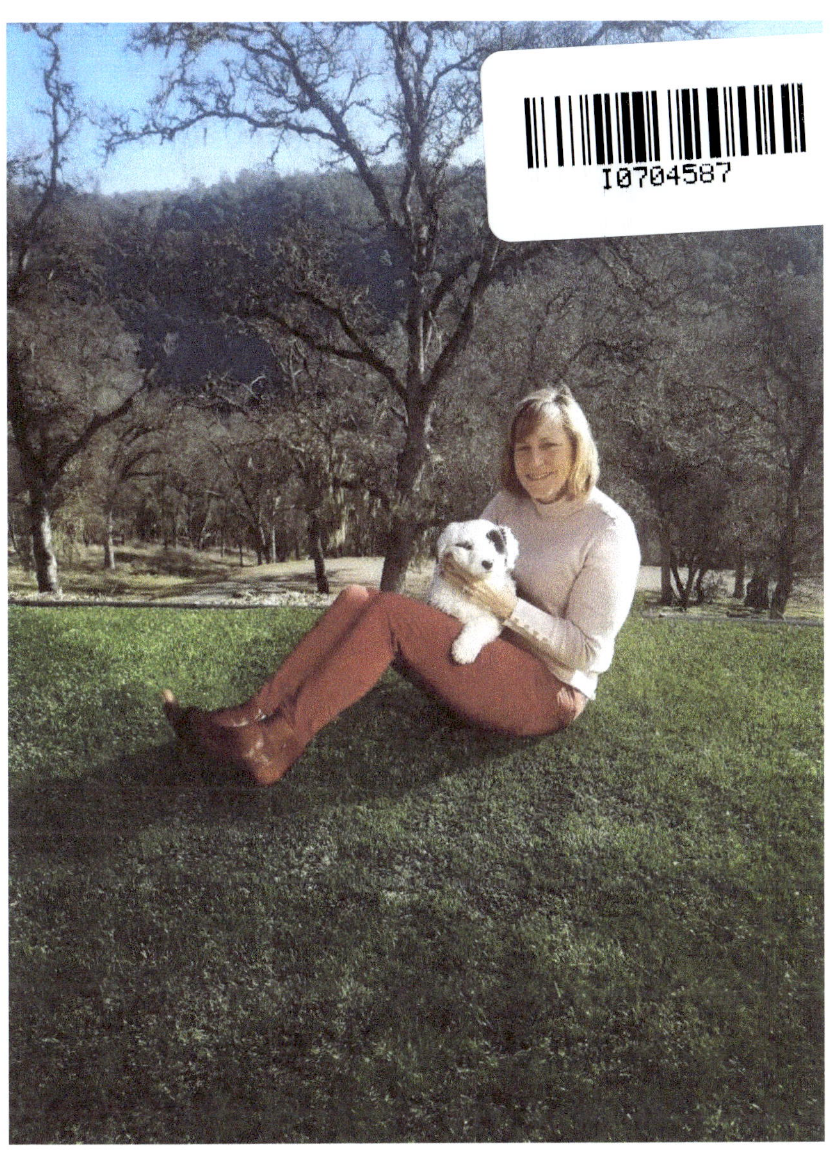

Dare to Dream – Again

My Breast Cancer Journey with Dani

ISBN: 9798339780038

Independently published

Dedication

I am dedicating *Dare to Dream – Again* to my mother, Nancy 'Kathryn' Ware. She was affectionately called Dani by my father Phil. She battled breast cancer in 1996 and spent the rest of her life encouraging others in their battle.

With great love, I dedicate my book to my children, Jason Wolfe and Shannon Cunningham. When I was first diagnosed, Jason, a Major in the U.S. Army, was deployed to Korea. He was able to email and call, and upon returning in July, came to California for a surprise visit. Shannon spent many hours sitting with me at the Kaiser Oncology Ward. I so appreciated her willingness to be with me.

 I am truly blessed with my children, grandchildren, and the rest of the family who lovingly supported me through my cancer journey and subsequent writing of this book.

Acknowledgements

To my four breast cancer sisters: Alisa, Cindy, Sabrina, and Nanette, a heartfelt thank you. They are all survivors of different types of breast cancer and showed me love and support in many various ways. From gifts of blankets, bracelets, and late night telephone calls, I was able to endure. My neighbor Cindy was ready at a moment's notice to visit or just to hear me "complain". She told me I was her first breast cancer friend since her recovery and that it was very emotional to see me go through what she had just experienced.

Thank you to my tennis friends from Fair Oaks Racquet Club and the Hangtown Women's Tennis Club. Their encouragement to see me back on the courts was deeply appreciated.

To the many friends who sent encouraging cards, emails, and offers of any assistance I may need. Thank you!

Many hours were spent at Coffee Republic in Folsom, CA, where owners, Ken and Renee Kremesec and daughters Madison and Mary Meyer, provided a space to be creative. The atmosphere was quite conducive for writing, plus the coffee and brownies are exceptional.

The beautifully designed rocks from Sacto Cali Rocks provided inspiration in telling my story. Thank you for giving encouragement to all of us going through cancer treatment.

Last and possibly most importantly the medical staff from Kaiser Permanente Hospitals: Roseville, Rancho Cordova, and Morse Ave. Thank you for making this journey bearable.

Table of Contents

About the author

Stephanie Wolfe Zimmer graduated from CSU, Sacramento with a degree in journalism and a minor in criminal justice. She later acquired a Secondary Teaching Credential in history. Stephanie is a former business owner and has co-authored two books: *Autumn's Cathedrals* with her son, Jason and *Kathryn's Kitchen* with her mother, Nancy. Currently she is a substitute teacher and is active in tennis.

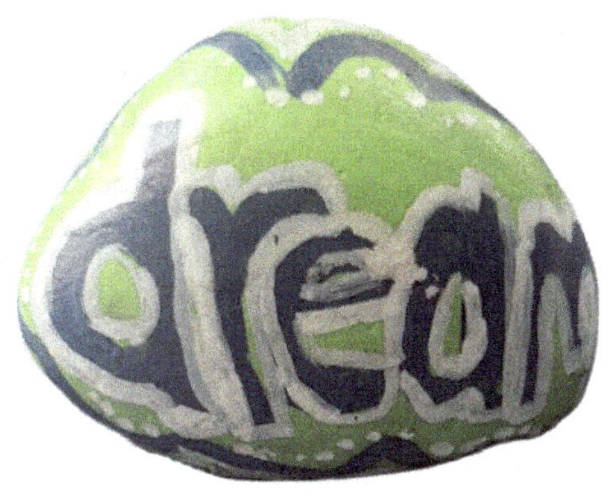

"I have gone thru the fire, emerged whole,
only to dream again!"
Author - Unknown

"Is it bad news?" I asked. "It is not good!" replied the radiologist. On, January 10th, 2019, those words were spoken to me, which set me on a five-year quest that would forever change my life. A routine mammogram, January 3rd, led to tests, scans, surgeries, chemotherapy and radiation - culminating with reconstruction surgery in 2021, fat restoration in 2022, and ultimately a nipple tattoo in May 2024. This is my journey, unique only to me, but certainly not any more important than the thousands of women and men who first heard their own "bad news."

During cancer treatment I hadn't considered writing a book about my journey. I actually felt like I was living in a fog and that I wouldn't be able to remember this period in my life. It was hard for me to journal so I thought that having lots of photographs would help me in the future to process what I experienced. About a year after my treatment, while weed-whacking on our property, I thought to myself how grateful I was to be healed and to have a future to pursue any goals and dreams I had. It wasn't until 2022 that I actually put pen to paper (fingers to computer). Now, two years later, I have finally completed one of my dreams, to write another book.

 I will share a little history of how breast cancer was discovered and the people who were instrumental in diagnosing and discovering new methods in treating patients. I will describe how modern medicine has evolved and what resources are available. I will also give current statistics published by the American Cancer Society. This is by no means a medical journal – just one layman's description of breast cancer history and medical terms.

From notable women in history, to my mother and myself, you will read of our accounts: first fear, then determination and finally embracing courage in battling this horrible disease. It is my hope that our stories will give insights that may help future cancer patients in their road to recovery.

If a picture is worth a thousand words, then an album is priceless. I will attempt to convey my story using photos, quotations, and the decorative rocks I acquired during my chemotherapy treatments. Accompanying me on my journey is Dani the dog, who joined our family just nine days before it was "never the same". With the support of family, friends and the incredible medical staff at Kaiser Permanente Hospital I have emerged to "dream again".

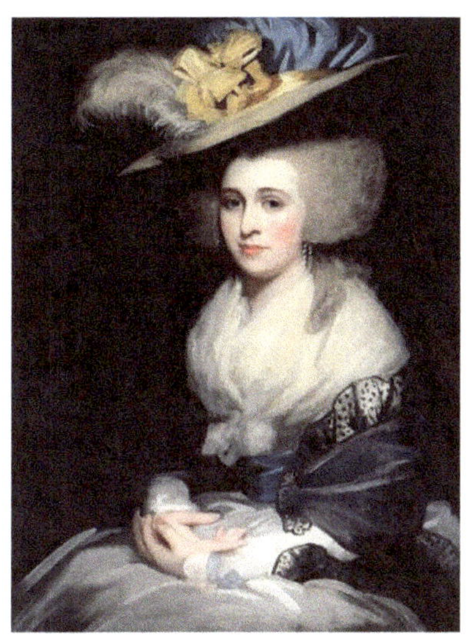
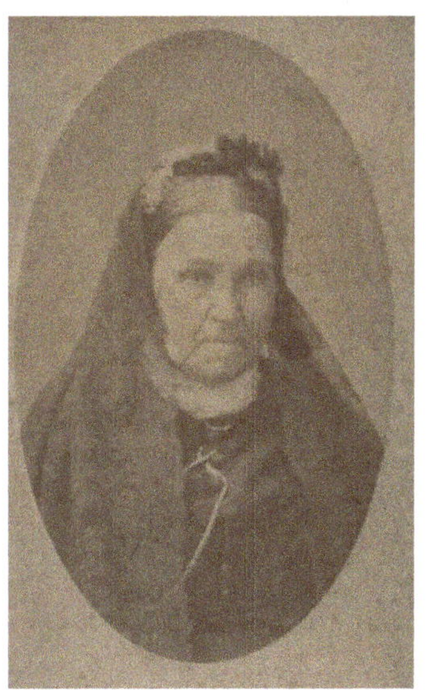

Abigail 'Nabby' Smith 1765-1813
Courtesy of Adams National
Historical Park, National Park Svc

Lucy Goodale Thurston 1795-1876
Wikimedia Commons Domain
Public Domain

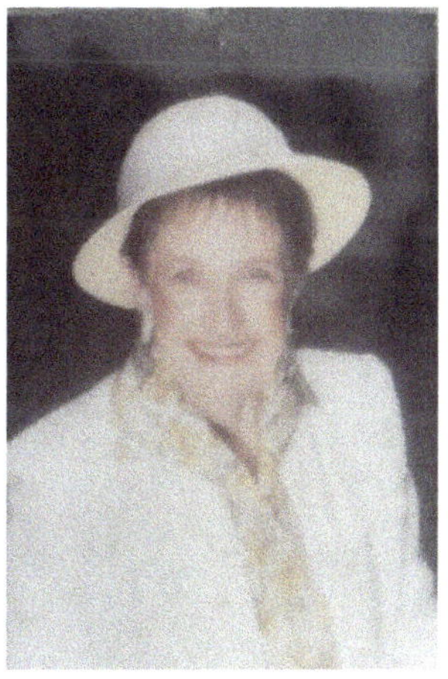

Nancy 'Kathryn' Ware
1930–2013 Private Collection

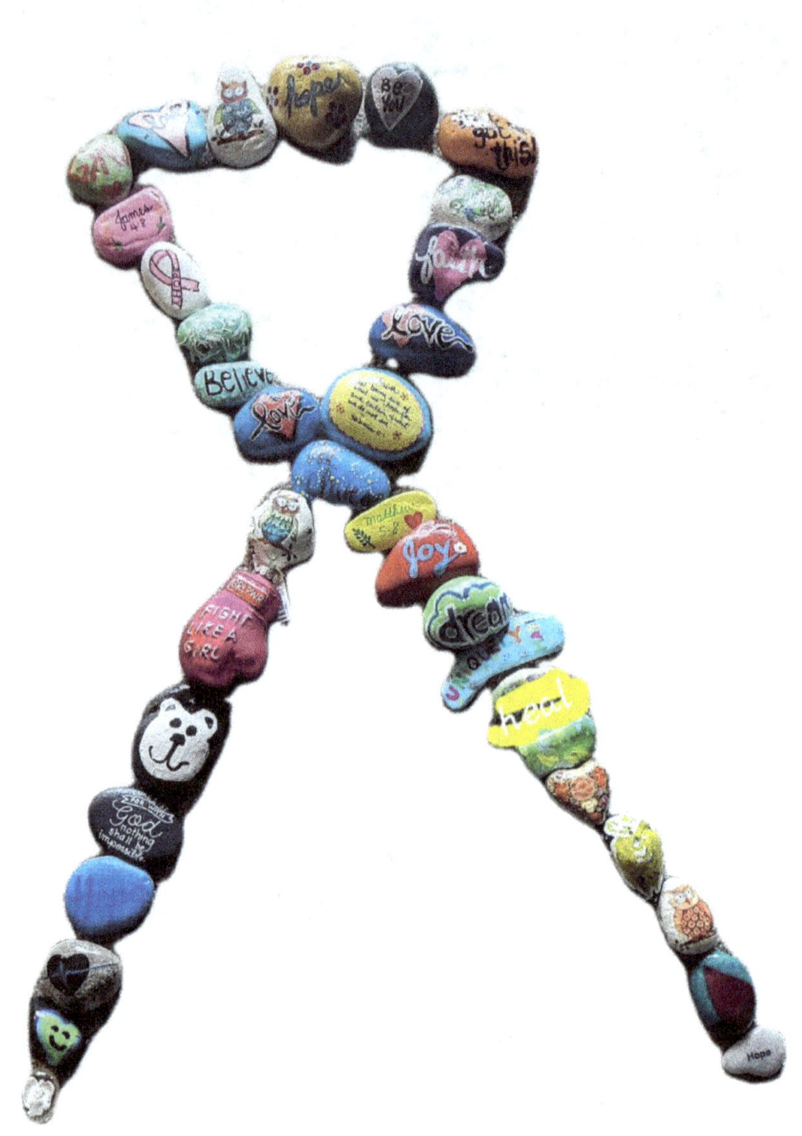

"When pain is unbearable it destroys us;
when it does not it is bearable."
Marcus Aurelius

"From her account of the moving state of the tumor, it is now in a proper situation for the operation. Should she wait till it suppurates or even inflames much, it may be too late… I repeat again, let there be no delay in flying to the knife. Her time of life calls for expedition in this business, for tumors such as hers tend much more rapidly than cancers after 45, than in more early life. I sincerely sympathize with her and with you and your dear Mrs. Adams in this family affliction…"[1]

Dr. Benjamin Rush, a noted physician and a signer of the Declaration of Independence, wrote to John and Abigail Adams in 1811 encouraging them to relay this devastating news to their daughter Abigail 'Nabby' Adams Smith. Nabby was the eldest of the four children born to Abigail Adams, July 14, 1765, in Braintree, Massachusetts. It was in 1810 at the age of 44, when she first discovered a lump in her right breast, thus, beginning her incredible ordeal.

Breast cancer in the 1800's was considered a dreaded disease, but Nabby like so many others in her era, was busy raising a family and running a household on a small farm in western New York. She sought advice and treatment from local healers, and potions but still her lump increased in size. In June 1811, she returned to Boston with her family to seek further guidance. In fact, she was told that, because of her general good health, she wasn't in any immediate danger. She was prescribed hemlock pills which were to "poison the disease".[2]

Nabby wrote to Dr. Rush describing how her tumor was getting larger and was "movable", and not attached to the chest wall. He felt that because of the position of her tumor she was a better candidate for surgery, reducing the chances of a reoccurrence or spread of the cancer. In his letter to her parents, he elaborated on the urgency of undergoing a mastectomy and the thought "of the consequences of procrastination".[3]

Nabby was willing to go through with the operation but first she had to gain her husband William Smith's approval. At that time, a woman did not have the right to make decisions on her own. Smith was in denial of the severity of her health, and went to libraries to educate himself. He finally agreed and the operation was scheduled for October 8, 1811 at the Adams' home in Quincy, Massachusetts.[4]

Dr. John Warren, Boston's most skilled surgeon performed Nabby's mastectomy without anesthesia. His son, John Collins Warren, (who in 1846 was part of the first public demonstration of a surgical operation using ether anesthesia), and other physicians aided with the operation.[5] Dr. Warren had prepared the family of what to expect, which for early 19th century was not pretty. There were no actual details recorded of the procedure but Olson (2002) writes, it is assumed that her family was by her side. Her dress unbuttoned to expose her right breast, the operation began. She was belted to a reclining chair, another physician held her right arm above her head, then Dr. Warren thrust the two-pronged fork deep into her breast. With a large razor he completely severed it. The tumor was larger and more widespread than thought, so he razed the lymph nodes under her arm as well. He then used a red-hot spatula to cauterize the bleeding wound.[6]

The whole operation was performed in less than 25 minutes. Her surgeons were amazed how stoically she endured the pain.

According to her father, she never cried out once. Nabby was weak but suffered no post-surgical infections. She stayed with her mother for over seven months before returning to her home in May 1812. Shortly thereafter she started having headaches and complaining of pain in her abdomen and spine. Her local doctor attributed to her malaise as rheumatism, which eased her anxiety. By spring of 1813, Nabby's health had declined considerably; her cancer had returned.

She told her husband that she wanted to die in her father's house. Travel arrangements were made and Nabby endured a painful three hundred mile carriage ride before reaching her parent's home in Quincy on July 26th. Her parents were shocked at their daughter's gaunt and emaciated condition. Abigail was so distraught and fell into a deep depression and was unable to even visit with her. It was John Adams who tended to his daughter during her final days: feeding, cleaning, and comforting her. Nabby died, August 15, 1813, just 22 months after enduring her mastectomy. In a letter to Thomas Jefferson, John Adams described her as being "a monument to Suffering and to Patience".[7]

"Thus instructed, and everything in readiness, Dr. Ford looked me full in the face, and with great firmness asked: "Have you made up your mind to have it cut out?" "Yes sir." "Are you ready now?" "Yes, sir; but let me know when you begin, that I may be able to bear it. Have you your knife in that hand now?" He opened his hand that I might see it, saying, "I am going to begin now." [8]

In 1855, Lucy Thurston age 60 underwent a mastectomy without any anesthesia under the care of Dr. Ford. In a letter to her daughter, Mary, dated October 29, 1855, she described in detail the procedure and subsequent healing.

Lucy was 23 years old when she and her husband Asa, left Massachusetts to become the first American missionaries on the islands of Hawaii. In her 40's she suffered from having had paralysis (most likely polio) that would later result in her doctor not recommending the use of chloroform as an anesthesia for her mastectomy operation. In late August of 1855 it was decided to "use the knife" and within weeks her tumor rapidly appeared close to the surface of her left breast which possibly could lead to become an open ulcer. An immediate operation date was set for September 12th. [9]

Lucy relied heavily on her Christian faith as she prepared for her ordeal and had her Bible and a hymn book nearby. In her letter to Mary, she described in detail the room where the surgery took place and the procedure itself. It was in a grass-thatched cottage, furnished with two lounges and a reclining Chinese chair where she sat during the procedure. A table was set up that held the instruments, strings for tying arteries and threaded needles used for sewing up the wound.

With her left arm extended back, her right hand grasping the chair, and her feet pressed against the foot of the chair, Dr. Ford proceeded to slice both sides of her breast. Her son Asa and daughter Persis were present ready to restrain her if needed and to provide her with cordials and other aid. After nearly an hour and a half, her left breast was cut out as were the "glands" (lymph nodes) beneath the arm, along with tying the arteries, stitching the wound and applying the bandage over adhesive plasters.[10]

 Lucy wrote in her letter that she felt she suffered nearly as much after the operation as during the surgery. For days she was fed teaspoons of chicken soup and a little wine. Within four weeks of the operation she was able to ride in a carriage with her husband Asa, who devoted himself in helping her recover. Lucy eventually was able to resume her missionary work and lived an additional 21 years.

"I woke up the morning of my operation feeling relatively calm. I took two pieces of masking tape and placed them over my breasts. The left read 'leave Eleanor alone'. The right side read 'farewell Mariah, I will sorely miss you' ".

On October 15, 1996, my mother Nancy 'Kathryn' Ware underwent a mastectomy to her right breast. She was 66 years old, a retired school teacher, a hospital volunteer, a writer and an overall busy lady. Mostly she was a wife, mother, and grandmother, whom her family adored. Her story is best told in an essay I found after she passed away and after I had finished my breast cancer journey. I wish I had read it earlier.

'It was the middle of August, 1996 while lying in bed that I felt a rather small lump in my right breast. I thought it could be a Neurofibromatosis tumor. I have suffered with NF my entire life and have small fibromas all over my body. I decided to just keep a check on it.

On August 28th I had a doctor's appointment for another matter and asked him to check my breast. He decided to check the tumor with a needle to see if it was a cyst. He then scheduled me for a mammogram, which to me feels like they are putting your breast through an old fashioned washing machine wringer or a fancy pasta machine. I sneakily tried to find out what the results were, but the technician deftly avoided my inquiry.

A few days later the medical clinic called and an impassioned voice informed me that I was to undergo an ultrasound. The date was Friday the 13th, which I generally hate and try to stay home, if possible. I nervously kept my appointment and unlike a mammogram this procedure was absolutely painless. I was getting concerned as clinics don't just do testing for the fun of it. I tried to engage the technician into a friendly conversation, hoping she just might let something slip. Being the professional that she was, she told me the results would be turned over to the radiologist.

That afternoon my doctor called to tell me I was scheduled to meet with a surgeon September 27th for a biopsy. Now I was really becoming frightened. Trying to keep my odd sense of humor intact, I named my breasts. The left one was to be called Eleanor and the right, Mariah. I have names for just about anything and everything.

It had been a long time since I had any surgery so I purchased a small tape recorder to listen to music during the biopsy. The doctor wouldn't allow it, explaining that I needed to respond if I felt pain when he excised the cyst. The procedure was relatively painless and the results were sent to the pathologist with an **Expedite** order. Now the panic set in. I spent the following weekend in limbo, trying not to think the worse. Monday afternoon, my doctor called.

"How do you feel?" he asked. I replied that my incision itched. "I'm sorry to tell you, the tumor was malignant and it is about 1 ½ centimeters in size". "Oh horse pucky", (actually she was more graphic), were the first words out of my mouth. "What do you mean? I have cancer?" Then I literally went into orbit, babbling to the doctor that I was too busy with my hobbies, working the local precinct on Election Day, and planning my next travel adventure.

He calmly told me to come in the following day and bring whomever I wanted, to discuss the next step. I asked if I could bring my dog - that was a no. It was like fate that my daughter, Stephanie, called me later in the day to see what the doctor had to say. I told her that I have cancer but said, "Don't tell Dad, this is something I have to tell him." I was debating how to break the news to my husband, Phil. When he walked in the door, all I could say was that I have breast cancer. He immediately took me in his arms and said how very sorry he was and how much he loved me. When I rested against his broad chest, I knew that this man would do anything in his power to protect me against anything and anyone that would hurt me.

The next day, we met with the surgeon. He assured me that the tumor was small and gave me the option of having a mastectomy or a lumpectomy which would only remove the cancerous lump, followed by radiation therapy. I was sent home with a pamphlet to read and a week to make a decision. I was in a state of shock, this couldn't be happening to me. I called the Cancer Society and talked with a support person. I was told I could get a second opinion which I did and chose the second doctor as my primary physician as he was familiar with neurofibromatosis and had an Irish name.

Phil and I discussed the options after reading the pamphlet. I felt because of my age and not being too well endowed, I would opt for the mastectomy. My loving husband assured me that he would love me whether I had two, one or no breasts. Also, having heard horror stories about radiation therapy and the amount of time it takes, was another reason for my choice.

The date was set, October 15th. Now I needed something to focus on. I was to be the inspector at the upcoming presidential election and our backyard was being landscaped. I tried to direct my thoughts on what to plant. I guess I still felt that if I didn't think about the cancer or surgery, it would all go away.

I had talked to people who had been through this procedure and found I was not alone. Statistics showed that one out of nine women will have breast cancer. Of course, I never thought I would become a statistic. I even contacted a local breast cancer survivor group and one women, in particular, knew I was under a great deal of stress and kept close tabs on me until the day of surgery.

The night before my operation, I fell apart and spent over an hour in my husband's arms sobbing and sobbing. It suddenly hit me that I was going to lose part of my body and there was nothing I could do, unless, of course, I refused to have the surgery and face a more horrifying way of life.

I woke up the morning of my operation feeling relatively calm. I took two pieces of masking tape and placed them over by breasts. The left read 'leave Eleanor alone'. The right side read 'farewell Mariah, I will sorely miss you'.

We went to early mass and then to the hospital. I had hoped Phil and Stephanie could be with me until I was wheeled away to surgery. But no, I was plucked out of loving arms and taken away to a holding area. The only thing I could take with me was my teddy bear and a mini tape recorder. I was now both angry and scared. I was finally given a tranquilizer and before I knew, the surgery was over and I was back in my room, groggy but, oh, so very glad, to see my family.

I was grateful, in that I could stay one full day in the hospital before going home. It seems to me that going through such an ordeal it should be mandatory not to be sent home right away. I was in pain and quite uncomfortable especially with two drain tubes coming out of my chest attached to plastic bottles.

I came home feeling much the worse for wear. I still had the feeling that this was not happening to me. Several days passed before I saw my surgeon and got the results. I had done a lot of praying and hoped I could accept whatever news was given. I was so very fortunate. The cancer was not invasive, nor was cancer found in the lymph glands.

I urge women of all ages to check your own breasts and if you find even the smallest lump, run not walk to your nearest doctor. Thank you, Lord, I am one of the lucky ones.'

Nancy, whom my dad affectionately called Dani, actively spent her remaining seventeen years writing a cookbook, *Kathryn's Kitchen*, becoming involved in breast cancer support groups, and participating in the Susan G. Komen fun runs. Some of those ladies became her dearest friends. I attended a few of the functions that were put on by her group and was amazed at the comradery shown by these survivors.

I always supported my mother, but actually never had any inkling what she battled. It wasn't until I was diagnosed with breast cancer at the same age, 66 years old, that I could finally identify what she went through. Part of me wishes she were still alive at that time to give me support. Knowing my mother, she would have been my biggest cheerleader. The other thought I have is I am glad she didn't have to see me go through this trial. Some survivors will say, watching another person walk this path brings back many painful memories.

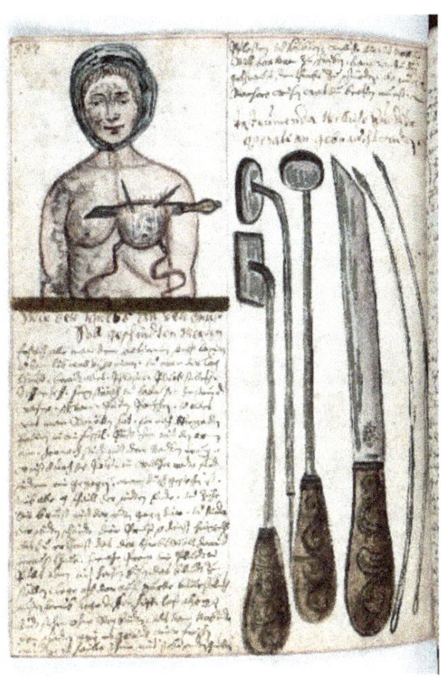

Breast operation and instruments used. Wellcome Collection

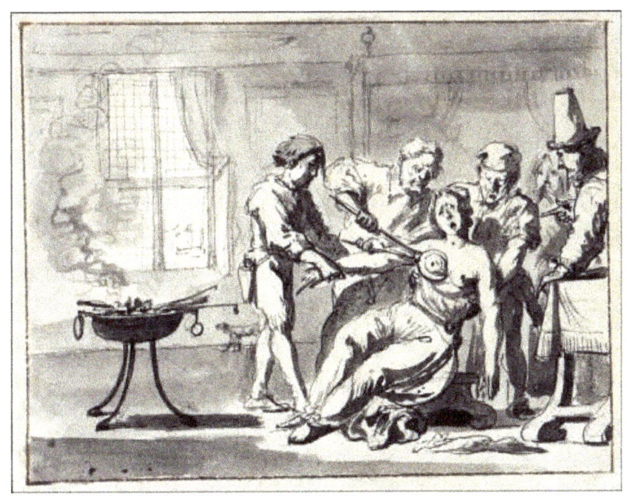

A 17th Century mastectomy. Wellcome Collection

"It is during our darkest moments that we
must focus to see the light."
Aristotle

"She had a tumour on her breast, after sometime it burst and spread considerably. As long as it was small she concealed it, and from delicacy informed no one of it; when it became dangerous, she sent for Democedes – a famous doctor of medicine and showed it to him."[11]

The Greek historian Herodotus (485 – 430 BCE) wrote about Atossa, daughter of the Persian King Cyrus, and her account with what was believed to be the first recorded case of a tumor in the breast. In his book, *Pathology of Tumours*, R. A. Willis quoted the writing of Herodotus who is known as the first historian in Western Civilization. Willis stated that Democedes purportedly cured her, but no further evidence was revealed.[12]

The earliest accounts of breast surgery dated as far back as 3,000 BCE and 1,500 BCE in the Edwin Smith Egyptian papyrus. Smith (1822 – 1906) was an American antiquities dealer who purchased the medical papyri in Luxor, Egypt. The papyrus was an ancient Egyptian textbook which described several cases of tumors and ulcers removed by cauterization and a tool known as a fire drill. The unknown author also "concluded that a bulging breast tumor was a grave illness, but the Egyptians struggled to treat it with cautery, knives, and salts, as well as adding arsenic paste which became known as 'Egyptian ointment'."[13]

Hippocrates, father of Western medicine (460 - 370 BCE), adhered to the "humoral theory of medicine". He believed that the health of the body was a balanced level of four humors: blood, phlegm, yellow bile, and black bile. He wrote that a bloody nipple discharge was the result of an excess of black bile within the body.[14] It was from him that the term cancer came, *karkinos*, a Greek word for "crab". He described the tumors as having tentacles, like the legs of crabs. The terms *carcinus* and *carcinoma* that describe non-ulcer and ulcer forming tumors were also used.[15]

Galen of Pergamon a Greek physician, (129 – 216 AD) born in modern day Turkey, further espoused the humoral theory and described "the therapeutic effects of releasing the black bile from the body".[16] He felt that some tumors were more dangerous than others and that breast cancer affected the whole body, so surgery wasn't necessary. He believed in medicinal therapy and prescribed medications such as opium, castor oil, sulfur, and salves. Galen was credited with using the word *oncos* a Greek term in describing a swollen tumor.[17]

Physicians throughout history had varied notions of what was the underlying cause of breast cancer. From the "humoral theory of medicine", to tight clothing, to the lack of sex (reproductive organs may decay), and to vigorous sex which could lead to lymphatic blockage were just a few. Many other tales such as curdled milk, childlessness, and mental disorders were often thought to be the basis of breast cancer. Also there were many differing ideas on how to treat the disease.[18]

During the 19th century in the United States, many surgeons performed operations based on their own knowledge and techniques. More information was learned about lymph nodes and their part in spreading the disease. In 1894, William Halstead became known for the "Halstead radical mastectomy" which surgically removes the whole breast, lymph nodes under the arm, and chest muscles under the breast. The following year, Wilhelm Conrad Rontgen a German mechanical engineer and physicist discovered the X-ray that ultimately led to the beginning use of radiation as a treatment option and developing the mammogram. He later earned the first Nobel Prize for Physics in 1901.[19]

In 1976 an American surgeon, Dr. Bernard Fisher, initiated a study comparing the effects of a radical mastectomy to that of a lumpectomy. He also adhered to the premise that the "addition of systemic used, adjuvant chemotherapy or hormonal therapy provided a survival advantage over surgery alone". This led to testing of tamoxifen that could prevent breast cancer. [20]

By the 1960's and 1970's chemotherapy was used as an adjuvant therapy alongside radiation after surgery to destroy any remaining cancer cells. It was during WWII that the Navy and Army studied troops who were exposed to mustard gas, which showed toxic changes in their bone morrow. They worked with compounds that would fight cancer of the lymph nodes. Eventually scientists discovered aminopterin, an amino derived from folic acid. It was used in the 1950's as a treatment for pediatric leukemia. Today there are many variations of the chemotherapy drug and treatment plan used in the cure of breast cancer.[21]

In the mid 1990's less than ten percent of women with breast cancer had a mastectomy. The development of hormone treatments, surgical and biological therapies and early detection from a mammogram allowed patients alternative care. Scientists also isolated genes that cause BRCA1, BRCA2, and ATM that have led women to re-think preventive care.[22]

History has taught us that some form of breast irregularities, (carcinoma) have been prevalent dating back to ancient times. Due to visible signs, (unlike internal cancers) lumps found in later stages of the disease allowed physicians to record their findings. We see from early documents, (papyri), and writings from noted historians (Herodotus and Hippocrates), to present day researchers, the diagnosis of breast cancer has evolved from ominous to a promising prognosis. Earlier, women were less apt to bring attention to any abnormality they found due to societal norms. Today there are multiple sources that are dedicated to researching, treating, and caring for breast cancer patients.

The symbol of pink ribbons, fundraisers and a month dedicated to breast cancer awareness are prevalent in treating this disease. In October 1985, the National Breast Cancer Awareness Month began. It was a partnership between the American Cancer Society, (ACS) and the pharmaceutical division of Imperial Chemical Industries to promote mammograms. It was helped along with First Lady, Betty Ford, a breast cancer survivor herself, in bringing more recognition.[23]

The pink ribbon is one of the most universal symbols used to bring attention to breast cancer. Charlotte Haley in 1991 first created a peach colored ribbon in honor of family members who had battled breast cancer and to raise awareness of the lack of federal funding. In 1992 Haley was approached by Alexandra Penney, Editor-in-Chief of *Self* magazine, with an idea to form a partnership. Haley felt it was too commercial and declined the offer.[24] This rejection led to the formation of a pink ribbon alliance between *Self* magazine and Estee Lauder, guest editor of the first year's edition of the Breast Cancer Awareness Month issue in 1991. She also was a breast cancer survivor. The objective was to distribute pink ribbons to Estee Lauder store locations in New York City then expanding nationwide.[25]

The most recognizable breast cancer organization, also incorporated the color pink. The Susan G. Komen Foundation was founded in 1982 by Nancy Brinker in honor of her sister who passed away in 1980 from breast cancer. The foundation's most notable fundraiser is the Race for the Cure. In 1983 the first race was held in Dallas, TX with 800 participants.[26] The logo design featured "an abstract female runner outlined with a pink ribbon". The logo was used until the early 1990's when the breast cancer survivor program was first launched. Pink became the designated color and the pink visors were given for survivor recognition. In 1992, the Komen foundation adopted the pink ribbon that was from the *Self* / Lauder alliance. In 2007, the Susan G. Komen Breast Cancer Foundation became Susan G. Komen and created a specially designed logo which included a pink "running ribbon" that is currently used.[27]

Breast Cancer is the second-leading cause of death in women in the United States second only to lung cancer. In 2024, the American Cancer Society (ACS) estimates 310,720 women will be diagnosed with invasive and 56,500 with non-invasive (in situ) breast cancer. An additional 2,790 men in the United States will be diagnosed with invasive breast cancer.[28] There are other types of breast cancer along with various treatment plans that each patient will undertake. If you find yourself as one of the statistics, there are many organizations and support groups to aid in your recovery.

When I was first diagnosed, it never occurred to me to take pictures. I have always kept a journal of my life events. It was not until after my reconstruction that I dared look at the photos and realized that God spared me. I am so grateful to be a survivor and it is my hope that you can find humor and inspiration from my journey with Dani by my side.

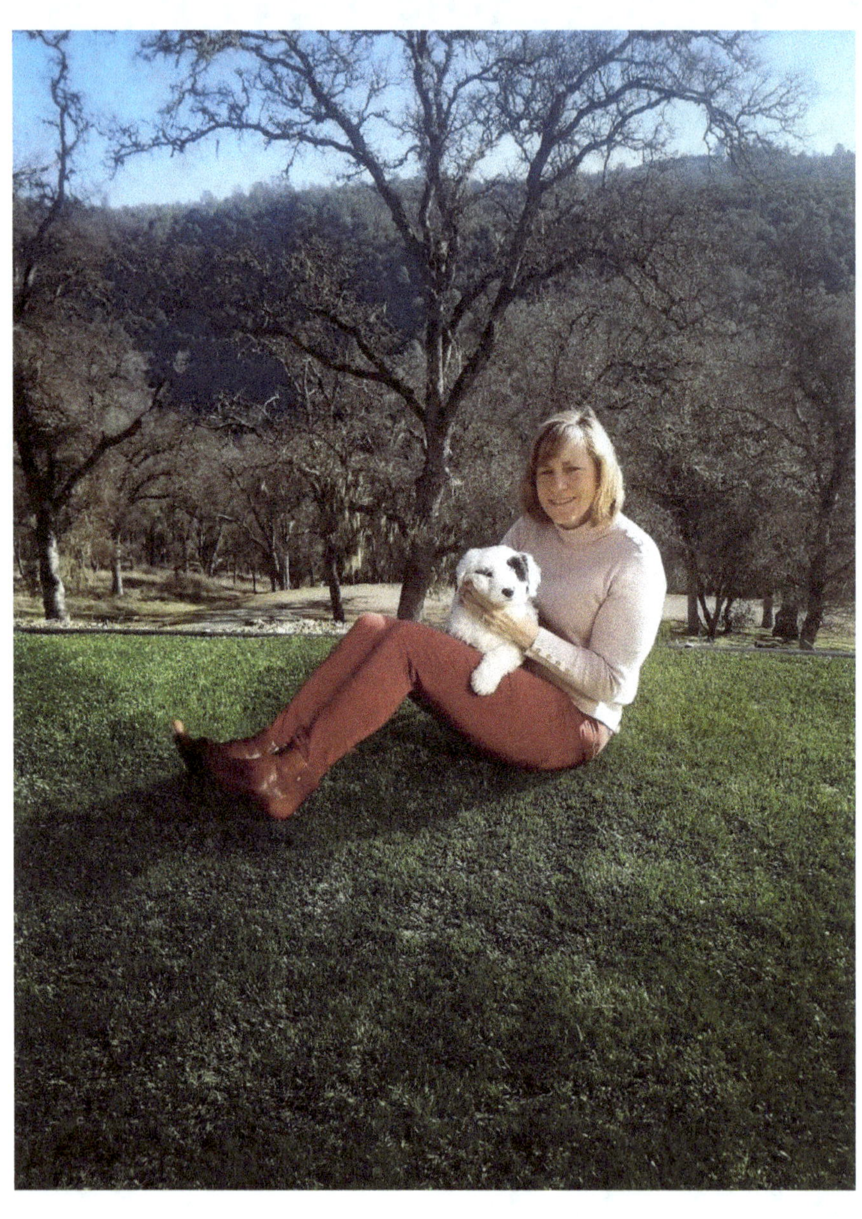

December 30th, 2018 – Unaware, playing with Dani

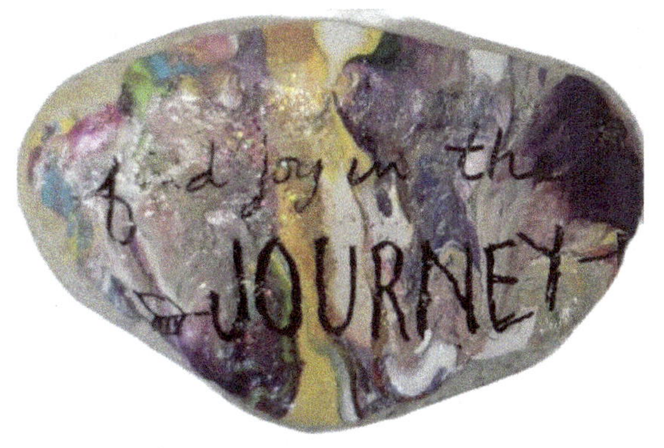

"I can do all things in him who strengthens me."
Philippians 4:13 RSV

It was Thursday, January 3rd, 2019, when I went to Kaiser Hospital in Roseville, Ca. to have my routine mammogram. As in the past I never gave it a second thought after having this procedure. The following Monday I received a phone call asking me to come back the next day to have another mammogram. It was a gloomy overcast day with light rain in the forecast. I recalled the weather as I was to play in a tennis match that evening and had things to do to get ready. After having the test I was sent down the hall to have a sonogram. It was told to me that I needed to undergo a biopsy and it could be done within the next two hours. I said that I would prefer to wait later in the week as I wanted to play that night. The nurse told me that it was in my best interest to have it done that day.

Well, I acquiesced, called the captain of the team, Alisa, and told her I might not be up to playing because I was scheduled for the biopsy. She immediately said, "Oh, No"! She had recently finished her breast cancer treatment and urgently convinced me to do the procedure ASAP. I still didn't think much of it. I called my husband, Nick and told him I would be detained and not to come down as there was nothing to worry about. Later in the day I left the hospital feeling fine but disappointed as our tennis match was canceled due to the rain.

I am by nature a person who upon hearing the possibility of bad health news for a family member, says a prayer then goes about my life believing they would be healed. I was soon to become someone who was not so nonchalant when faced with my own disturbing news. It was 11:00 a.m., Thursday, January 10th. I was sitting in my car waiting to go inside for a piano lesson, when the phone rang. It was Kaiser Hospital and the radiologist asked me when I would be home? I told her around 3:00 p.m. I then asked if it was bad news and she responded, "It is not good"!

I was numb, I couldn't process what I just heard. I called Nick to tell him to be at home by 3 o'clock. He suggested instead for me to come by the tennis court as he was giving lessons. I responded with a resounding NO and said this could be the worst news I will hear and I wanted to be at home. After canceling my piano lesson, I drove to a local store to pick up merchandise. I wanted to kill time. It is so hard to put into words the feelings I was experiencing. To me, those four hours were the most fearful and traumatic time I felt during my cancer journey. I remember walking aimlessly around wishing I was in a hole or could cover my head with a hood. I wanted to bury myself and not think. As I looked at other people, I thought how carefree they seemed. Is this what it means to know you are dying? I had often wondered how people who hear devastating news from their doctor react.

I was in tears as I drove home. All I could think of was how to tell my family I had cancer. I had just celebrated my 3rd wedding anniversary the day before and thought how sad Nick would feel. I couldn't even imagine how the rest of my family would respond. I called my neighbor Cindy who was a breast cancer survivor. She calmed me down and said I probably do have cancer but I am not going to die. She asked if I wanted her and her husband, Mike to come over to support me when I get the phone call. I said yes.

When I arrived at the property, Nick was already home and Mike and Cindy came shortly after. We positioned ourselves around the kitchen counter and waited. Precisely at 3 p.m. the radiologist called. She said, "You do have breast cancer, (Invasive Ductal Carcinoma, Stage 1), and it is treatable." I literally collapsed against the counter and said, "Thank you, Lord". I was told that the surgery department would contact me soon to inform me of my options. I can say that having others be with me to hear the diagnosis was awesome. This experience was all new to me and I am forever grateful for Cindy and Mike's support during this time. Little did I know where my journey would lead me that year. I underwent three surgeries, two rounds of chemotherapy, twenty five radiation treatments and moved into my own apartment after separating from my husband!

When something dramatic happens to you, it is natural to think about how your life was before. In my case, ten days earlier we brought an adorable puppy home. Dani (who I named after my mother) is a half Portuguese Water Dog and Border Collie. The book cover picture was taken the day after we adopted her when she was only seven weeks old. I was so excited to have her and really had not a care in the world. I felt healthy: actively playing tennis, substitute teaching, and working at two wineries. Life was great!

That was then, now I had to concentrate on all the necessary procedures and treatment I would undergo. I cannot express the care and professionalism that Kaiser Permanente Hospital gave me. The following day after hearing from the radiologist, the surgery department called. They said that I had "invasive ductal carcinoma with lymphovascular invasion. Estrogen receptor positive, Her2 negative - Stage 1A". The long diagnosis described meant nothing to me except the words Stage 1A. I was told I was treatable and all would be good. They set up an appointment with the surgeon for ten days later to discuss my options.

Now the hard part was before me. How to tell my family without disrupting their lives? I called both my son, Jason, and daughter, Shannon, assuring them that my breast cancer was caught early and was treatable. Of course, they were worried for me but sensed I was handling it well.

The next few weeks were first spent consulting with my surgeon, Dr. Reid Towery. I opted for a lumpectomy as my tumor was determined to be little, 1.8 centimeters to be followed up with radiation. I also continued with my tennis, teaching, and winery work. Ironically, at one of my winery jobs, I attended a meeting where we had to share something with other employees a fact they didn't know about us. It had only been recently I was diagnosed with cancer. This exercise was intended to create a bond with fellow workers and I felt it wasn't the time to unload my "bad news" as most of the stories were uplifting. I did share that I play tennis and with my partner, Luda, our Fair Oaks tennis team won a tournament at Indian Wells several years earlier. Ultimately, my employer, along with family, friends, and co-workers became an integral part in supporting me in my cancer journey.

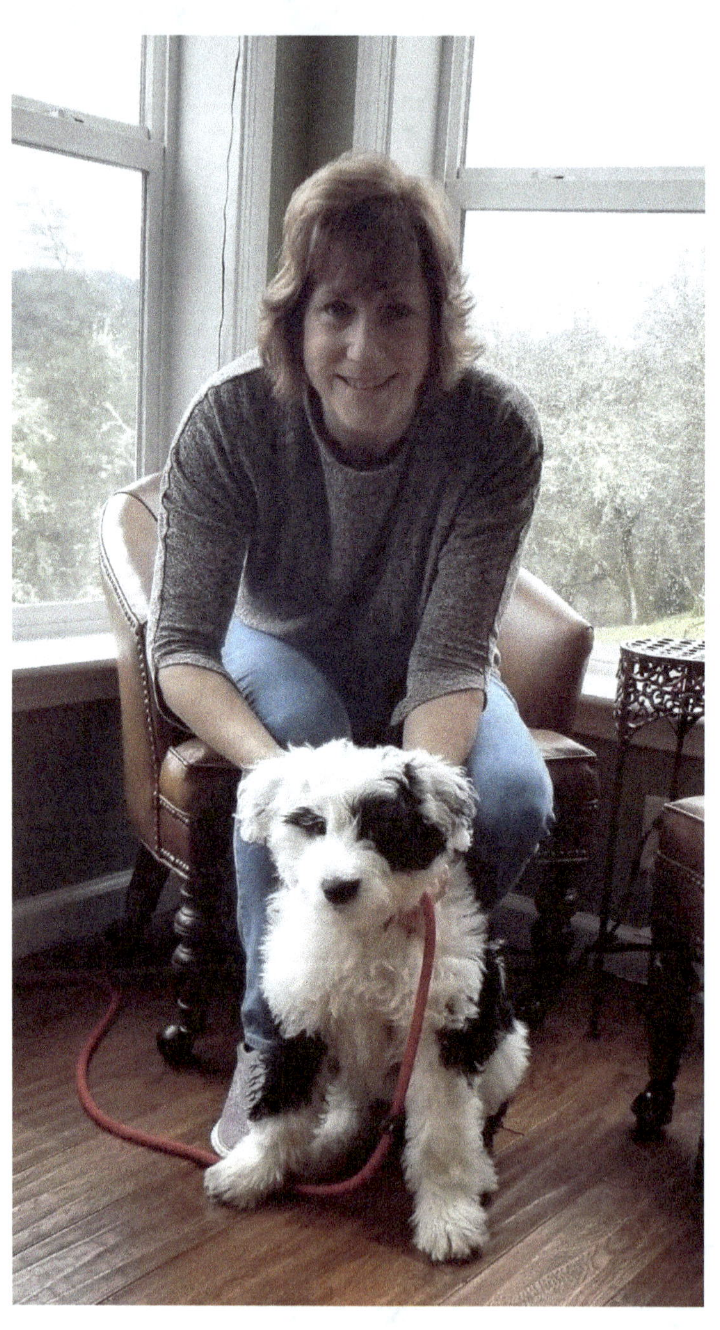

January 30th – Lumpectomy ready to go

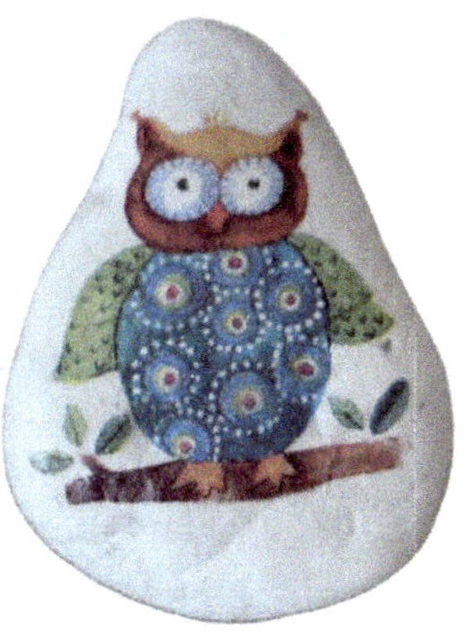

Reflecting back to the day of my first surgery, January 30th, 2019, nothing notable stands out. I had to look at pictures to remind me of how I looked and, possibly, be able to describe my thoughts. The night before, I had gone out to dinner with my husband and prepped for the following day's surgery. I do recall thinking about my mother's breast cancer surgery and getting strength knowing how well she recovered. Actually, the Owl Rock that I acquired from one of my chemotherapy sessions reminds me of her. Nothing else significantly comes to mind other than making sure I had set aside what was needed to take to the hospital. I wasn't scheduled to spend the night as this was considered a routine lumpectomy. I did sleep well, not overly concerned at all for what I was to undergo.

The following morning I got myself ready and played with Dani. By then she was a 12-week-old pup and was the joy of our family. Once I was admitted to the hospital, I had some time before I was to enter the operating room. My husband, daughter, and other family members came in to express their love and said they would see me later. I do recall that I felt very calm and really wasn't concerned about anything. After all, the doctor told me my cancer was treatable and everything would be fine.

My surgery lasted for several hours. The next thing I remember is a nurse in the recovery room explaining to my husband that the surgery went well **BUT** the tumor was bigger than originally thought, (4.8 cm) and the sentinel lymph node was found to be positive. The sentinel lymph node is generally the first lymph node where cancer cells spread from the primary tumor. During a breast cancer operation the surgeon uses a harmless dye and a very minimal radioactive solution to locate and remove the nodes to have them biopsied. It was also discovered that my cancer may have spread to more of the chest wall.

I was still in a fog-like condition and didn't comprehend the severity of my health condition. After another hour or so I was released to go home and was told that the surgeon would be calling soon to again tell me my options. I do recall not feeling any pain and there was no nausea associated with the anesthesia. Nick took me home and settled me in on the couch. Other than needing to be helped into the house and keeping Dani from bouncing on me, I was relaxed and feeling fine. After a short amount of time I regained my appetite and proceeded to enjoy a light meal.

Within a few days, I felt normal other than looking in the mirror at my chest (which wasn't very well endowed) at a one - sided flat figure with scars. I continued with my usual activities and waited for Dr.Towery to call. I don't think I was overly worried or really concerned about the future. This was all new territory for me but I felt secure in the knowledge that my cancer was treatable and curable. The phrase "ignorance is bliss" best described my outlook. I've since asked friends to recount how my demeanor was during my cancer treatment. One friend said I exhibited a "matter of fact" attitude in the early stages of my journey.

A week after my surgery, I was informed of the extent of the findings from the lumpectomy and sentinel lymph node biopsy. I do recall having feelings of anxiety of the unknown. I still had faith in my doctors and tried not to anticipate my future. Again, I have never been in this situation dealing with a serious illness for myself or a family member. To me, my mother's breast cancer was far removed from my reality. As I mentioned previously I had no concept of what she was feeling until I read her account years later. She never complained and felt fortunate that having a mastectomy cured her cancer. The premise that one doesn't really know how life's misfortunes feel like until it happens to you, is "spot on".

Another week passed and I was to meet with Dr. Towery again. This time I had my daughter, Shannon and dear friend, Robin (who was a retired surgical nurse), accompany Nick and me to the consultation. I think I was in a state of denial of the severity of choices I would need to make in my upcoming surgery. Ultimately, it would be my decision on what course of action to take. Having Robin present was helpful as she could - if asked - give me her objective medical advice.

It was during this timeframe the beginning cracks to my marriage were surfacing. Nick and I had only recently celebrated our three-year wedding anniversary. My illness was new territory for both of us to maneuver. Looking back, I realize that I acted and reacted in ways that were not typical of me. That is not an excuse, just reality. I have never had any major health issues to deal with other than the occasional illness that was common and minimal. I think Nick did his best in supporting me physically and probably felt I didn't need other's input for my treatment. Our communication skills were never the best and this situation certainly didn't help. For all my independence I now realize I needed more emotional support from my spouse and didn't know how to articulate it.

I did decide to have a full mastectomy along with removal of additional lymph nodes under my right arm. The day before surgery, I was taught how to care for the tubes that would be inserted during the lymph node removal. This part of the procedure would actually prove to be the most uncomfortable and painful. February 21st brought on my second surgery. Like my first operation, I was surrounded by family and emerged with no glitches nor side effects. I was able to leave the hospital the same day somewhat tired but once settled at home, felt fine. For days I had to drain the tubes and measure the amount of bloody lymph fluid that came out. A week later my tubes were removed as the lymph fluid had stopped draining. Fortunately I did not develop lymphedema, a condition where swelling of the arm occurs after removal of lymph nodes. Once the tubes were taken out, the pain began.

By this time I was spending more nights with Dani in the spare room due to my restless sleeping and dealing with unknown emotions. I remember researching on the internet, stories of other breast cancer patients and their experience with tube removal and was surprised to find that I was not alone in feeling pain. The actual taking out the tubes did not hurt but for a few days after, my chest was very sore. It was probably during this time that I took more pain medication than after both of my surgeries where I only required minimum doses of OxyContin. I definitely feel very fortunate and blessed that my surgeries were relatively easy and uneventful compared to others.

During this period I was scheduled for genetic testing. The findings showed no known pathogenic (disease causing)

mutations or variants including BRCA ½. It was suggested
that neurofibromatosis (NF) could be one explanation for my
breast cancer since my mother was a carrier. I also entertained
the thought that because I had been negligent in getting
routine mammograms, this could be a contributor. There was a
gap of a few years that I failed to be checked. I did not dwell
on this fact, as this would not be helpful to my mental well-
being. There was nothing I could do to change the past. Now
all we were waiting for was the pathology results from the
second surgery.

 It was the end of February while walking the property,
Dr.Towery called with the news. He told me there were 9
lymph nodes of the 17 removed that were cancerous and along
with the original sentinel node being positive, 10 out of 18
was the final count. I didn't ask if that ratio was bad. There
was certain information that I wanted to avoid knowing as
there was nothing I could do about it. I do recall asking him
what my cancer stage was now rated. I held my breath praying
that he wouldn't say Stage 4. After what seemed like an
eternity, he said I was assessed a Stage 3A. He went on to say
he felt they had removed any remaining cancer that was in my
chest wall. The next step would be receiving a call from the
oncology department to set up further treatment options.

March 6th was the day we first met with Dr. Manpreet Kaur
Sidhu who would become my most trusted ally in this journey.
I'm sure that most cancer patients will acknowledge that their
oncologist plays one of the most important role in their
treatment. She was no-nonsense, explained exactly what my
surgery revealed and what my future treatment would entail.
IF my cancer had not metastasized then I would be offered
"adjuvant (curative) chemotherapy with AC-Taxol, followed
by adjuvant XRT and adjuvant endocrine therapy". I had no
clue what she was outlining but I did catch the word **IF**. My
response to her was "**If** it has metastasized, am I a goner?"

  She did explain that if I had a metastatic disease – where the cancer has spread to either bones, liver, lungs, or brain - we would approach treatment based on the extent of the disease and that patients were known to go on to live many productive years. She said that I would be considered Stage 4 and there was even discussion of palliative care that could help me understand choices for further medical treatment. She ordered a PET scan for March 13th with a follow-up appointment the next day to discuss the results. According to Dr. Sidhu's written summary, "patient seemed quite overwhelmed at the visit". You think!!!

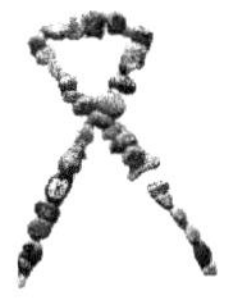

43

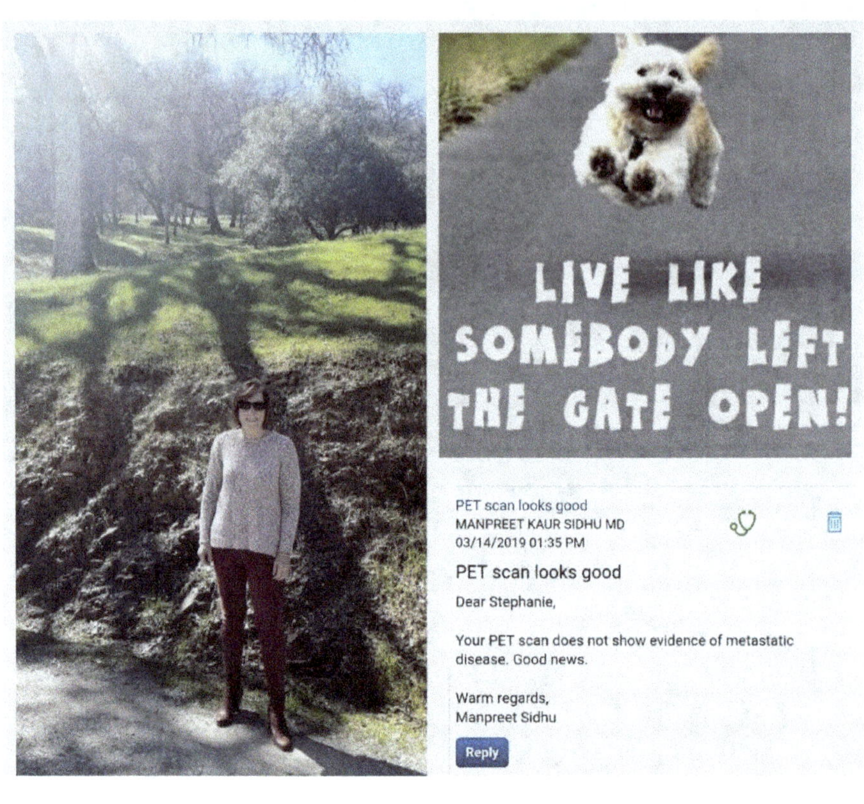

March 14TH - going to Kaiser to hear my fate

Encouraging poster in Dr. Sidhu's office (fundrazr)

Emailed PET scan report

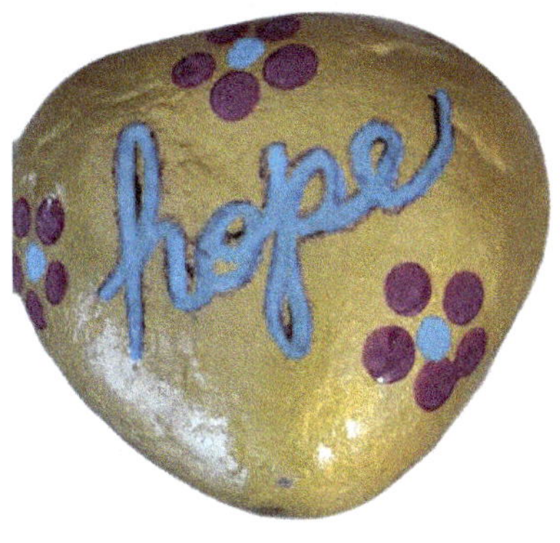

"We need hope, or we cannot endure."
Sarah J. Maas

I have no recollection of how I felt during the period before my PET scan. I chose to go alone for the appointment as no-one was allowed to accompany me inside. Looking back I realize that many of my tests and treatments I would go solo as I felt healthy enough and didn't want to be an inconvenience. Of course, I had numerous offers of support and for my chemotherapy sessions I generally was accompanied by family or a friend. The PET scan took about 25 minutes and I had to lay perfectly still. I remember feeling disoriented and not connected to my body. My mind had not comprehended yet what was going on inside of me. Other than having a one-sided flat chest, nothing seemed different. I didn't feel sick and certainly could not entertain the thought that I might be dying.

The morning of March 14th, I attended a ladies bible study at my church. Everyone had been praying for me. As I was leaving, one special lady came up to me and told me that the Lord spoke to her and said I would be fine. At that moment a peace came over me that to this day is hard to describe. I am a

Christ follower and know the power of prayer and that my future is already determined. I came home to sit with Nick and wait for the 3 o'clock phone appointment to hear my fate. When my follow-up consult from the PET scan was booked, we opted for a phone call instead of driving down to Kaiser Hospital which is an hour away. I do remember Dr. Sidhu looking a little perplexed but agreed to it. In hindsight it did seem odd to potentially hear devastating news by phone.

While at home waiting for the dreaded news, I did receive a phone call from the doctor's nurse, stating Dr. Sidhu preferred me in the office after-all to discuss the results. I thought this was not going to be good if she wanted me in person. As we readied to leave, I asked Nick to take a picture of me. I said that no matter what the tests showed, I felt healthy and would not believe any bad news. We were silent driving down and while walking inside the office I told him, "I feel like I'm in a western movie waiting to hear if the judge sentences me to hang." I know that I did not feel that same fear and panic I had while waiting for the results from my original mammogram back in January. I definitely had some anxiety and still remember thinking **why** do the nurses feel the need to take one's blood pressure every visit. My numbers that day were off the chart. I don't know what they expected!

We had barely settled in our chairs, when Dr. Sidhu breezed into the office saying, "I always want to start with the good news. Your cancer has not metastasized; the PET scan was negative". This was all said before she even sat down. Even as I write this my eyes are filled with tears, at the relief I felt hearing the news. I bent over in my chair and kept saying, "Thank you Lord". I guess I didn't realize how much stress my body was carrying. I later realized the PET scan result was emailed to me when the nurse called earlier that day - another reason to set my phone on for notifications.

Dr. Sidhu outlined my upcoming regimen, stressing this was not going to be a piece of cake. First I was to undergo a MUGA (multiple-gated acquisition) scan, a nuclear medicine test that reveals how much blood my heart pumps with every heartbeat. The results indicated that my heart was indeed healthy and strong to endure treatment. There would be a general information class that entailed living with cancer, chemotherapy protocol, and managing side effects: going bald, suffering with nausea, experiencing diarrhea, and feeling extreme weakness, etc… The class also addressed the necessity of having reliable transportation as a great deal of time is spent traveling to and from appointments. I was also scheduled for another CT scan, physical, and a 3rd surgery. I had the choice to either receive the chemo drug via intravenous therapy (IV) or have a port surgically implanted in my chest. I chose the latter as I could not imagine being poked numerous times in the arm.

I took a picture of the poster Dr. Sidhu had mounted on the wall. The dog appeared exuberant and acted as if it didn't have a care in the world. I would occasionally look at this photo as a reminder that one day I would be as carefree. My outlook in life had already changed beginning with my first diagnosis. I recalled thinking that l wasn't going to let this cancer beat me, not knowing what was ahead for me, but feeling so grateful for the chance to find out.

By the end of March I had concluded all necessary preparations and was ready to begin the battle in my healing process. April 1st my treatment began; this certainly would be no April Fool's joke.

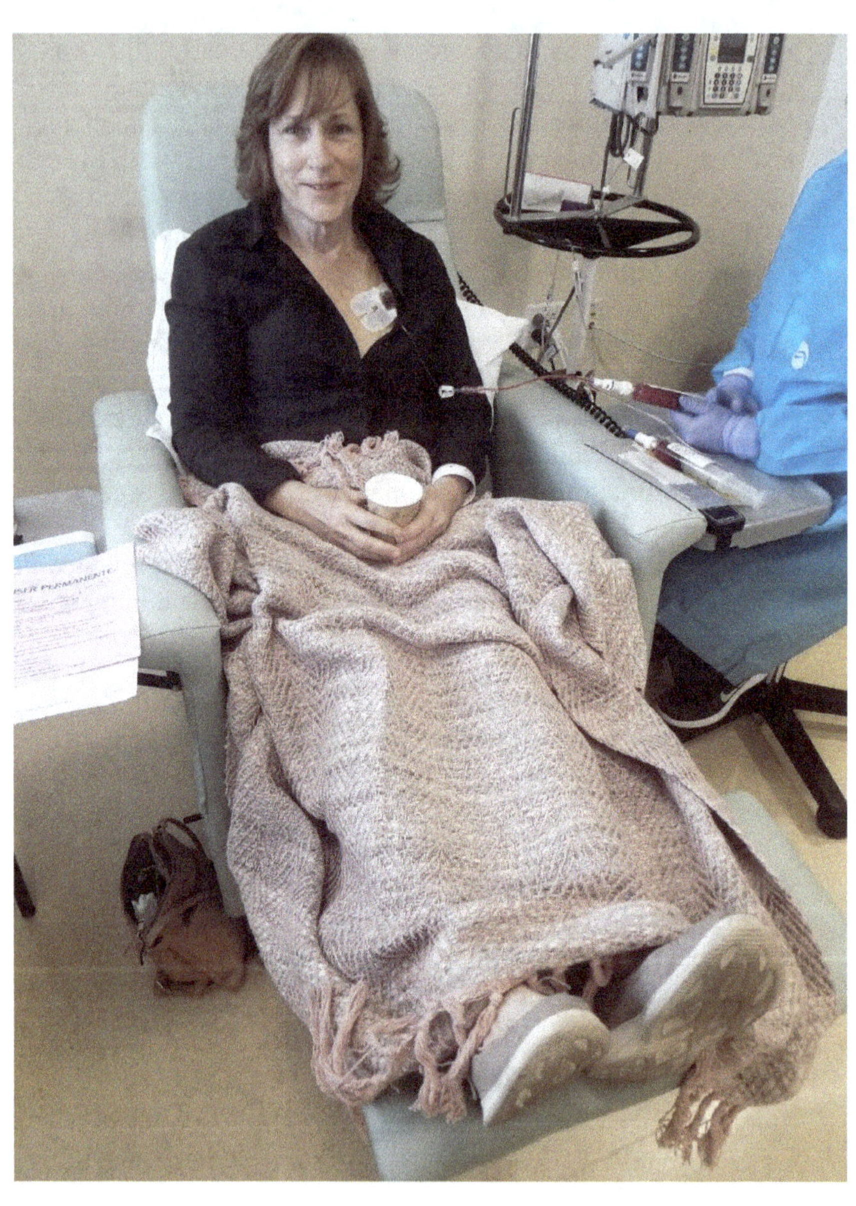

April 1st – First chemotherapy

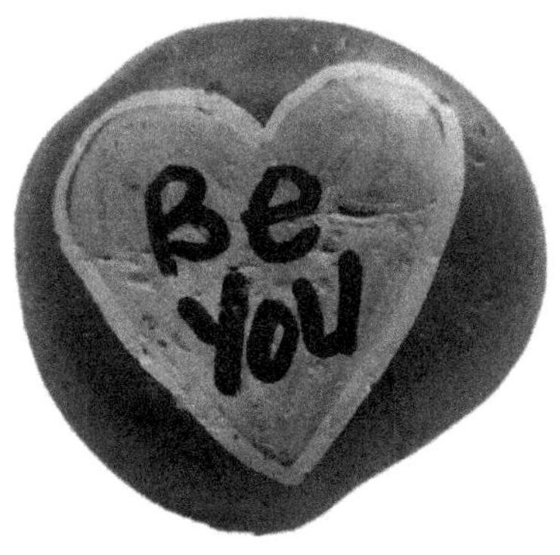

"Accept what is, let go of what was,
and have faith in what will be."
Sonia Ricotti

I would not consider myself a runner but I have completed a marathon in my 30's, 40's, 50's, and 60's. In each race, I had different strategies on how and when I would cross the finish line. The one thing that was common to all four races was the confidence I had, that I would not quit. In fact in my last race I was one of the remaining five people to finish. The point is, there was an end and I attained my goal. To even consider running a marathon was not on my list of must do's. I was 39 years old, my brother Dave was 40, when we thought it would be a "fun" thing to accomplish. For weeks we trained by increasing our mileage on runs and actually eating pretty healthy (sugar and carbs were almost non-existent). The day of the event came and we would see if all of our preparations were for naught. My goal was to run more than walk and finish with a pace under the five-hour mark. I did complete the event just past my intended time but still felt this incredible high that I did it. Dave also was elated as he reached his goal of finishing under five hours. Not everyone who started the 26.2 mile course would see it to the end.

I think of my cancer journey in terms of my completing a marathon. The big difference was I did not sign up for this event, it was handed to me. No matter the circumstances I had a goal to reach. It was nearly three months since I was first diagnosed. I had finished all necessary counseling, surgeries, and scans; it was time to begin the race.

The day before the start of my chemotherapy regimen, Nick and I went on a motorcycle ride, (I was the passenger). When faced with cancer, every moment seemed more precious to me and to be enjoyed. It was a beautiful sunny day and I felt peaceful and upbeat looking forward to beginning treatment knowing that once I started the sooner I would finish. I actually enjoyed that ride not feeling the anxiety that sometimes I experienced. I still consider myself a novice since my first time on a motorcycle was at the age of 62. We went to one of the wineries where I worked and were met with good wishes. Later in the day I had to go to Kaiser to have blood drawn which was part of the program I was to follow for the next seven weeks: blood tests, chemo infusions, shots, repeat.

My treatment plan consisted of Sundays having blood drawn before noon, then Mondays receiving a chemotherapy infusion of Cytoxan Adriamycin which is a highly toxic drug used to kill cancer cells in the body. Unfortunately, healthy cells are also eradicated. Decadron (Dexamethasone) a type of corticosteroid that helps decrease the immune system's response to cancer in lessening symptoms to allergic-type reactions, was also given. I would then skip a day and return the following five days for a Zarxio injection (Neupogen) in the stomach. This was to help reduce the incidence of infection and stimulate the growth of white blood cells. Several medications were suggested if needed: an antihistamine (Claritin) when taking Neupogen which also decreases body aches, Compazine (Prochlorperazine) for nausea and Ativan (Lorazepam) to combat anxiety or insomnia. The nausea and anxiety medications were the only ones I needed. I was then given a reprieve for six days, only to repeat the cycle. I was scheduled for four rounds of treatment beginning March 31st for a blood withdrawal and ending May 19th for my last shot. Two days later we would then board a plane to Atlanta, Georgia.

April 1st, while waiting to leave our home I wrote in my journal how nervous, anxious, and weepy I felt. I was concerned about the "unknown", how my body would react. I always want to be in control of my senses and was afraid that I would lose it by crying and throwing up. Reading accounts of other cancer patients who used the word "battling" in describing their journey, also scared me. I reminded myself that I had many friends and family that were in this fight walking along side me.

 Nick accompanied me to my first chemo infusion at Kaiser Hospital. When registering for the appointment the clerk handed me an envelope. She told me a lady left it at her desk and to give it to me when I arrived. Inside was a bracelet and an encouraging card. I was so overwhelmed and cried as the person who left it for me was someone I had never met, only talked with on the phone. Nanette is a neighbor to one of my dear friends and a breast cancer survivor herself. I was given her phone number as a contact person who would inform me about wigs and the best place to purchase them. I had only talked with her a few times and mentioned the date I was to begin treatment. She would become one of my four breast cancer sisters that I depended on in my journey. I actually never met her in person until four years later.

While waiting to be called in for treatment, I looked around the room and saw several women wearing scarves. Some had a person accompanying them; others came alone. I felt like I was a member of a select club and realized I wasn't alone in my cancer battle. One patient directed me to the bookshelf and said there was a basket of inspirational rocks that I could choose for each visit. I have over 40 of them as a reminder that I am a survivor. They have come in handy while writing my book. There were also knitted caps that were donated from some very caring ladies.

My name was called and we were escorted in. The area was set up with various stations, behind curtains or out in the open. Like myself, some patients had their full head of hair, some wore wigs, scarves, and or hats, while still others were comfortable in their baldness. I had never been in an oncology treatment room and was amazed to see how other individuals appeared while fighting their own battle not knowing the end result. One patient was softly strumming a ukulele and another was holding a little dog in her lap. Dani would definitely not be able to sit still so I actually had a stuffed replica made of her to bring to future treatments.

 A nurse directed me to my chair where I was made to feel comfortable. I was given a pillow and had brought my own blanket - a gift sent to me from Sabrina one of my four breast cancer sisters who underwent multiple challenges in her journey for survival. A nurse then offered me chocolate, graham crackers and an assortment of beverages: water, cocoa, or soda. This wasn't "happy hour" so wine was not listed as a choice. Instructions were given to what I might expect during this time. It was disconcerting looking at the tray beside me with vials of what appeared to be blood; it was actually the medicine. All I could think of was the poison that was to be inserted into my body. I knew it was meant to kill the deadly cells but would also eliminate some of my healthy ones. The procedure would only take about two hours. I was all settled in, the IV was inserted into my port and the

medication began to flow. The whistle sounded; my marathon
had begun!

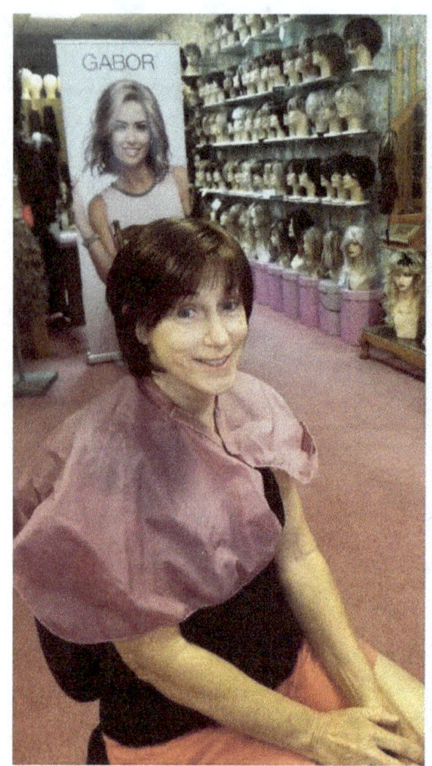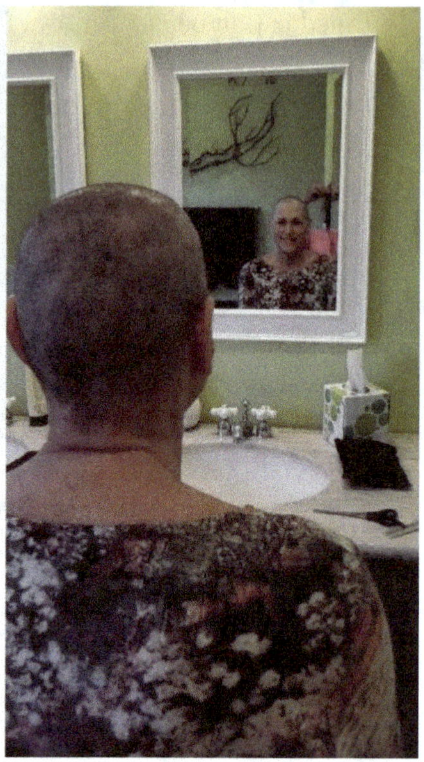

April 9th - Wig shopping / buzz cut

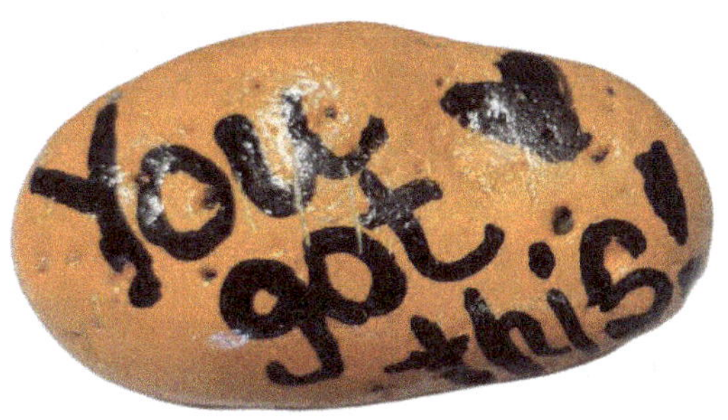

*"Press forward. Do not stop, do
not linger in your journey, but strive
for the mark set before you."*
George Whitefield

I was grateful that I didn't suffer many side effects from the
first infusion; in fact I felt pretty ok. I did take some Ativan
that helped alleviate the anxiousness I felt earlier and needed
some nausea medicine to settle my stomach. That week I spent
a lot of time commuting to the hospital (an hour's drive) for
my shots. During my reprieve week I did notice strands of hair
left in the bathroom sink and on the floor. By my 2nd infusion,
April 15th, my hair seemed much thinner and I knew it
wouldn't be long before I faced the razor.

My daughter, Shannon, came to many of my chemo infusions
and shot appointments. I appreciated her willingness to be
there with me even though I was fine being alone. I think that
family members of cancer patients have their own unique
struggles of how to be of help and also how to deal with their
fears of what may happen to their loved ones. Other friends
also came to the hospital to sit and cheer me on. I had my
beloved Dani at home to play with and decided to send a
picture to a company that made a reproduction of her. It was

so realistic that when I picked up the package at the post office, a lady wanted to pet my dog. I knew after a few hospital sessions, a stuffed animal wasn't very sanitary and left Dani Jr. at home.

Within a few days after my 2nd chemotherapy treatment I began to face the reality that my appearance was going to be altered and with that, I felt unnerved. I knew it was time to shop for a wig. My sister-in-law, Eiva (affectionately called Rah Rah), accompanied me in this venture. I had never been in a wig shop let alone put one on. I tried several, based on my hair color and length, and chose two quality hair-pieces. Now that I was equipped with my wigs and seeing more hair falling out, I was ready for my first buzz cut. I thought I would have more time because it was only a week after the second infusion.

 My neighbor Cindy volunteered to do the deed. I was so nervous and sat with my back to the mirror while she shaved me. When finished she said that I looked really good. It took me awhile before I would swivel around. I actually buried my face in my hands and kept saying, "I'm scared to look". At first glance, I thought I appeared like my brother Chris when he was younger and my grandson Tyler when he was little. I then tried on each of the two wigs I had just purchased. I didn't like how they looked on me, yet at the store I had been happy with my choices – later I realized my decision making could have been affected by the chemotherapy drug. Cindy loaned me her blond wig that she had worn during her cancer treatments. I liked the style and eventually donated my new wigs to the cancer society and only wore hers while at work or at special functions. I was comfortable donning a ball cap or a newsboy hat when going to appointments or running errands. At home I was more apt to wear a beanie or have nothing covering my head. The important thing was to be as comfortable as possible.

My first outing wearing the wig was Easter, April 25th. I was very happy with my new do. Rah Rah hosted the family which happened to be the last family event that I felt relatively normal.

In the early stages of the round-one infusions my feelings fluctuated from calm and happy to apprehensive and emotional. I was happy to have made the hair transition plans but wary of experiencing the possible extreme side effects of chemo. The nausea and vomiting while being completely bald was my biggest fear. I could not imagine myself in such an unpleasant situation or how I would look and feel. I did not know how to articulate my feelings and, subsequently, felt scared and lonely. In my spare room I spent a lot of time on the telephone with my cancer sisters and close friends. What was especially helpful was they would ask me how I was feeling. There was no judgement and the empathy and love they gave was truly appreciated.

Some days I felt pretty energetic; other days I was extremely fatigued and would sit on the couch most of the afternoon. In the morning I could do chores or work an early shift at the winery on weekends. Sometimes I would take a substitute teaching job but soon realized that I couldn't be effective in managing a group of students. I would not go back into the classroom until after my last radiation treatment. At times I felt exhausted, drowsy and sometimes confused in simple decision making. I was not accustomed to asking for help in simple matters such as fixing a meal, walking around the property, or dealing with a rambunctious puppy. In my mind I was becoming a burden because of my physical limitations let alone trying to get my emotional needs met. I described to others that I felt like I was living in a foggy state. In medical terms this mental change or cloudiness is sometimes referred as "chemo brain".

Dani was now 5 ½ months old and such a joy to have around, but being a puppy she still needed a lot of attention and discipline training. As much as I adored her, I was finding it difficult to do my part for her care. There was a time that I actually was willing to let her go because I couldn't embrace the thought that things would be easier. That was another instance where my decision making was influenced by the medication. I was feeling so overwhelmed and felt my only option was to relinquish her to another family. We actually had Dani's father Bento, a Portuguese Water Dog, come to the property. Ultimately, it was decided that Dani would stay even though I couldn't imagine how things would be different.

The last stages of the first round of chemotherapy brought on the complete loss of all bodily hair. There were some perks to this as I didn't need to shave my legs nor under my arms. Getting ready for the day was a breeze in that my scalp dried really fast. I had to look intently at pictures to see that indeed I had lost all my eye brows and lashes, which apparently I was okay with. I also experienced some Neuropathy (numbness and tingling of hands and feet). Thankfully, it was mild and eventually went away. There are a number of other side effects that can occur depending on the patient and type of chemotherapy used. For a long time the memory of a strong foul odor coming from my urine stuck with me. It reminded me of smells that emanate upon entering a nursing home and it was a constant reminder that my body was also sickly. I feel fortunate that I have not suffered any long term effects from my treatments.

Occasionally, I would work at the winery as I had a flexible schedule based on how I felt on any given day. I did stop working soon after an event that was held in early May at the local fairgrounds. It was a beautiful day and I felt almost normal as I performed my barista duties (pouring wine). Before I knew it, my energy level had suddenly dropped and all I could do was find a seat and pray I wouldn't pass out. This was the first time I felt I had no control over my body.

 I realized that I couldn't count on having the stamina needed to continue to work in any capacity. In fact, I almost requested to leave but decided to sit while my co-worker did the pouring and most of the talking. Looking around I thought how everyone looked so happy, healthy and enjoying life. A lady approached me and said she loved my hair and that my face had a beautiful glow to it. Wow, I felt so grateful for her kind words and started to cry. Not only was my body failing me, my emotions were going haywire.

After that day, I entered my reprieve week, then finished with my first round of chemotherapy the 3rd week of May. I did play in a recreational doubles tennis event only to withdraw after two rounds – what was I thinking? It takes more than a cancer diagnosis to keep us tennis players down. My body was definitely tiring out and it was time for me to just accept the bodily changes, maintain a positive attitude while avoiding any stressful situations, and to look ahead to the day I would be completely healed. Meanwhile I shifted my thoughts to flying to the East Coast for a week-long visit with family. Ironically, this trip was planned a month before hearing my "bad news".

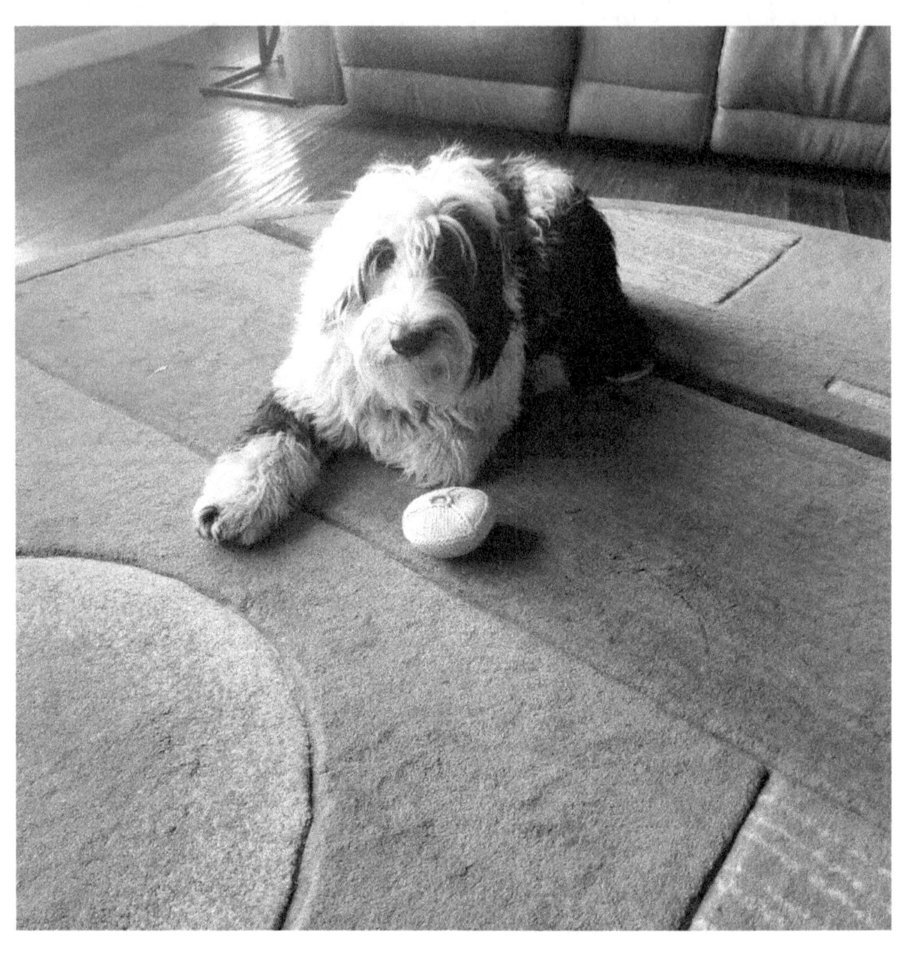

Dani watching over one of my Knitted Knockers

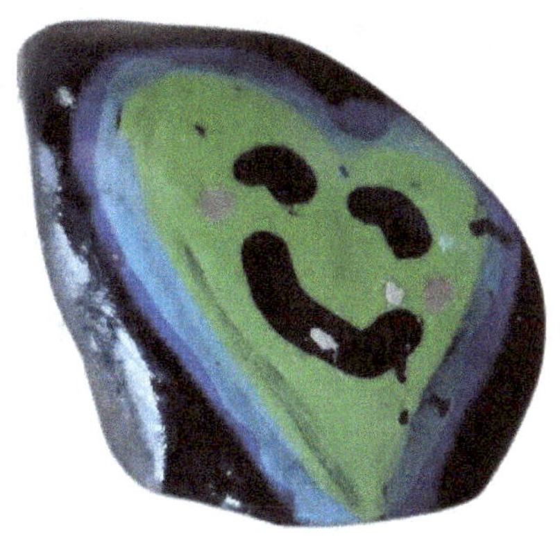

I never gave it a thought about how I would look in clothes, especially a bathing suit after my surgeries. The healing process required wearing loose clothing or post-surgery camisoles that have easy accessibility to care for the attached tubes and treating the wounds. When I was able to wear a bra, I was prepared as my sister-in-law, Michelle, made me several Knitted Knockers. They are a form of a breast prosthesis made using cotton yarn and have the shape and feel of a real breast. I had never heard of such a thing and was so grateful that Michelle took it upon herself to knit these. I started with four of them in different colors and ended up with two, as Dani liked to help with the laundry.

Eventually, Kaiser Hospital referred me to a local company who fitted me for a prosthetic bra and a breast prosthesis. All the swelling was gone from my chest and my incisions had healed. I was eligible every two years to replace the prosthesis if needed and yearly to receive three new bras. Wearing these garments gave me the confidence that I appeared normal to anyone looking at me. At my age (66) I had not even entertained the thought of having breast reconstruction and resigned myself that I would live the rest of my life with my one small breast. As long as I could eventually play tennis and lead an active life once treatment was over, I was satisfied.

Basically my wardrobe hadn't changed much. I had my new "under garments", wore looser clothes (as I had lost a few pounds) and covered my head with a wig or stylish hat. Packing for my trip was quite easy as I knew I would not be venturing out a lot. My oncologist gave the ok that I could travel if I wore a mask on the plane, rest as much as possible, and return within a week to begin the 2nd round of chemotherapy. I promised that I would adhere to all her advice and thanked her for giving me permission for this short respite. I couldn't wait to start my vacation, putting all thoughts of the oncology ward out of my mind and pretending I was as normal as other travelers.

First stop was Atlanta, GA. to attend a high school graduation. It was extremely hot and I became fatigued with even short walks. At times I would feel chilled and spent a great deal of time sitting outside to get warm. This bodily temperature change would be an issue later in my treatment.

One evening I was channel surfing and came across a documentary about a women who was dying of breast cancer. I couldn't take my eyes off the screen as she talked about her journey and lessons she learned in life. She said the most important message she could impart was to show love to your family and friends. After she died, her husband was interviewed and he made the statement, "When the doctors told us she had 5 lymph nodes out of the 25 removed, we knew she wouldn't make it." It was at that moment I truly realized that I had been spared as my count was 10 cancerous out of 18 taken. Some would think that would be a depressing show to watch, but as a believer I had the peace that indeed my life was in God's hands and my heart overflowed with gratitude that I could survive this. There are always the questions that cancer victims struggle with: why did I get this disease and why is my prognosis what it is?

 A few days later we rented a car and drove to South Carolina to visit my brother Andy and Michelle (the awesome knitter). It was during the drive I was beginning to feel extremely weary and my body felt like it was on fire. I also had an insatiable craving for grapefruit juice which I never had before. We eventually found a drugstore to get a thermometer and juice. The plan was if I had a fever we would go to the nearest hospital. Thankfully, my temperature was only slightly elevated so we proceeded on.

The few days spent in S.C. were uneventful, but soon I came to the realization that maybe I should not have taken on this venture. We did go on some short outings to restaurants and the beach, but it was evident that I didn't have a lot of stamina. It was great being around family but it was definitely time to head home. I was extremely tired and had to save my strength for round two.

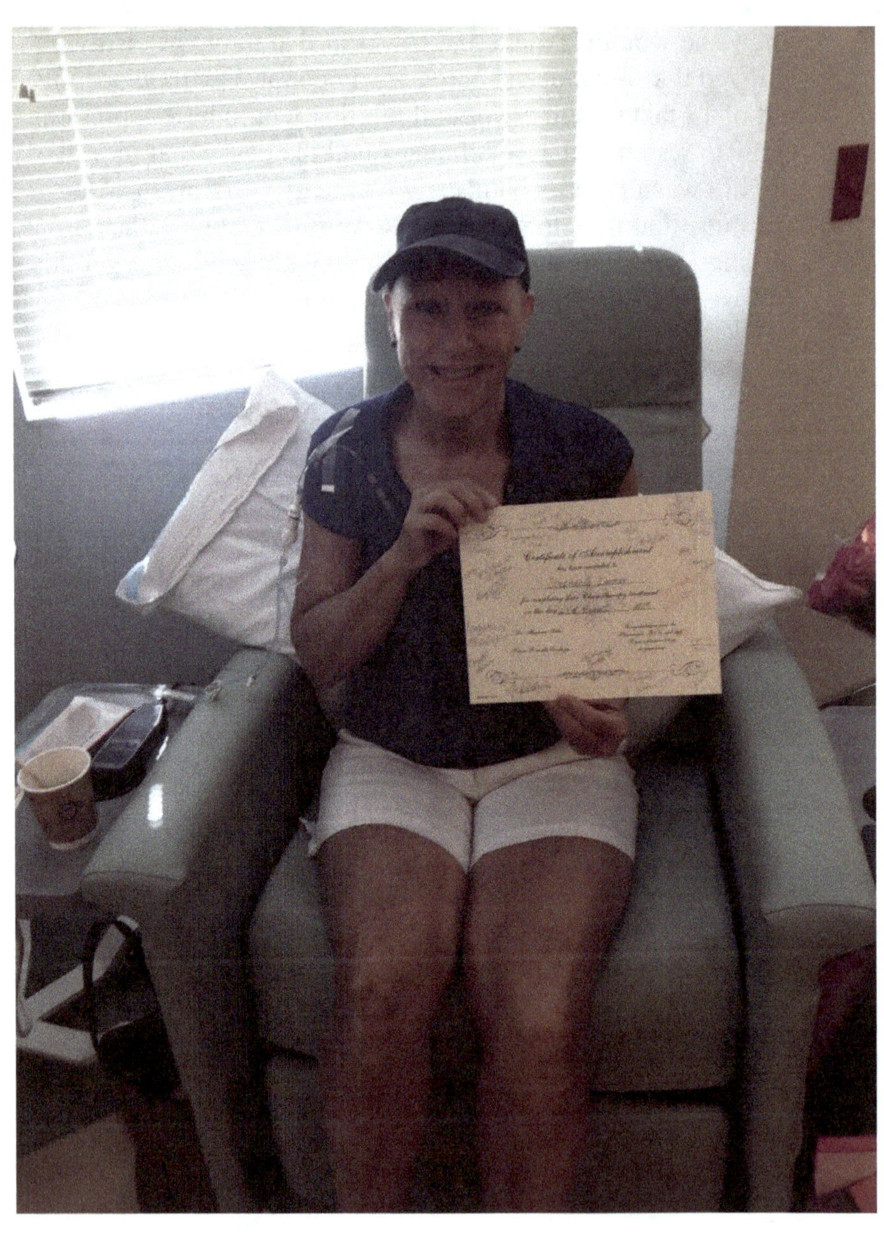

August 27th – Graduation from chemotherapy

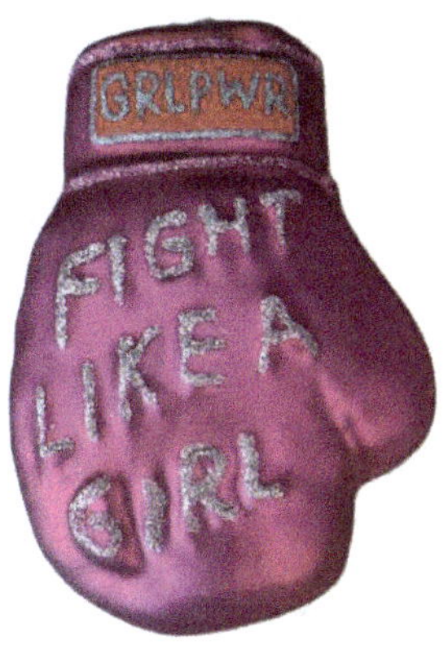

"Fate whispers to the warrior,
'You cannot withstand the storm'
and the warrior whispers back,
'I am the storm'."
Author – Unknown

We had only been home from our trip for three days when my second chemotherapy treatment began. It was Tuesday, June 4th, I was schedule for twelve sessions of Paclitaxel (Taxol). Every Monday I had to have blood drawn to check my white/red blood cells, kidney, and liver counts. I was able to drive myself for these procedures and the infusions were not as time consuming as the first cycle, lasting only 45 minutes. My routine was set for the next three months and I was looking forward to the end of August when all chemotherapy would end.

The medical staff in the oncology ward were like second family to me. The care and love they showed was indescribable. It was as if I were living in a bubble for months and felt protected while having treatment. In my mind, I had put my life in their hands, with complete trust in their care. Ironically I felt more at peace when I would go for my infusions than when I was home. Even now I can't describe why there was so much tension in my marriage. I know we argued a lot over seemingly little things. In hindsight, I realize I wanted and needed more compassion and empathy for my situation. I felt that I had to be strong and couldn't show any weakness nor vulnerability. What I desired, was at times to be held, allowed to cry and just express what I was feeling. Being the independent person I am, I found it hard to ask for what I needed. I also couldn't do my share of work or care for Dani. Not only were my emotions heightened, my body was going through more major changes.

Almost immediately after starting Taxol, I suffered with spikes in my temperature. I felt chilled and could not get warm enough. Most afternoons I would sit on the couch covered in a blanket. While attending church I would start by sitting inside then almost immediately retreat outside. I would put a chair next to the building, basking in the sun while listening to the sermon from an overhead speaker. After the service, people would approach me to ask how I was feeling or if I needed anything. I also recall other times the thoughtful gestures when people allowed me to go ahead of them in a checkout line or offer assistance in loading groceries into my car. These acts of kindness were so appreciated and sometimes brought tears to my eyes.

It was Sunday, June 23rd when I was admitted to Kaiser Hospital. I had been experiencing fevers almost daily ranging between 99 to 100 degrees. By the time I went to the hospital my fever had reached almost 103° degrees. Generally, chemotherapy patients are instructed to seek medical attention if their temperature is above 100.5° due to the fear of an infection that could lead to sepsis. I was immediately led to an examination room where various tests were administered. I recall the doctor expressing concern that possibly my heart had been damaged. At that moment I felt disconnected to my body, trying to shut out any conversation and telling myself this is not happening to me. If not for the effects of the medicine in my body, I still couldn't believe I had cancer much less experiencing a heart attack. I likened my thoughts to that of a Peanuts cartoon, where Snoopy heard conversations that sounded like a muted trombone, "Wha, wha, wha, wowah!"

Eventually, I was put in a room, hooked up to a heart monitor and given antibiotics. It was determined that I had a Neutropenic fever which is not that uncommon in a chemotherapy patient whose white blood cells are low and cannot fight an infection. Also, my troponin level (protein released into the bloodstream during a heart attack) was higher than the normal range of 0.04ng/ml. Tests revealed my levels were 0.51ng/ml.; thankfully, my body responded to the antibiotics in fighting any infection I may have had, and no damage to my heart was found. After four days I was released to go home and a week later resumed my chemotherapy infusions.

I found that during this time it was hard for me to write in my journal. It was easier for me to print out a monthly calendar listing my appointments and record any medical issues I had. I would also write a short memo of what I was thinking and feeling that particular day. This information helped me when I had visits to my oncologist and especially now when writing my book. I then would draw a huge X on the date which helped me visualize I was one day closer to finishing treatment.

One incredible entry in late July lifted my spirits immensely. My son, Jason, a Major in the U.S. Army, had just returned from a deployment in Korea. He was only home at Ft. Leavenworth, Kansas, for a few days when he decided to fly out and surprise me with an unexpected visit. That particular morning I was waiting for my daughter to come to the house to pick up my grandson Tyler. As I opened the front door, I couldn't comprehend that it was my son. It was like a scene on the news of a soldier returning home to surprise their family. I was dressed in shorts and a tee shirt with no hat, when he walked in and gave me a big hug. I hadn't seen him in over a year and I am sure seeing his mom bald was a little shocking. I was completely overwhelmed with this loving gesture and began to cry. I couldn't compute that he was really here. Thankfully my daughter was filming everything for this "Candid Camera" moment.

During the month of August I felt the most intense effects of the chemotherapy. I experienced elevated temperatures and extreme fatigue almost daily. I recorded many days where I felt sickly and weak with nausea and diarrhea. I also was feeling more sensitive, actually cried when I thought all my cancer pictures on the phone were deleted. Only four more weeks and the poison would end.

August 27th was celebration day as the last of my chemotherapy infusion was given. My husband accompanied me to the hospital where my daughter met us with flowers and a cake. It is the practice of the oncology ward to present a signed diploma with best wishes from my care team. I was happy and upbeat; now I could relax and recover in the next three weeks before undergoing radiation.

Actually the week following my last infusion, I suffered with even higher temperatures and tiredness than before. I waited several days before insisting I go to the emergency room to be checked out. After several hours of tests, it was determined that my body's reaction from all the chemo was an elevated fever and that I wasn't in any near danger of getting an infection.

I truly believe having the support of family and friends walking alongside helped me through this battle. There were several instances when my tennis friends would come to our home to visit and bring lunch; other friends would bring dinner. These were the moments that I could almost pretend to be normal. It is still hard to describe what I was feeling at this time. Friends have told me that I was upbeat about my prognosis but definitely appeared overly anxious and distressed in my home life.

 I had always been a healthy person and not one to succumb to being a needy patient. I was at a point where I was tired of everything in life being revolved around my health. I felt that I was losing control of how I would normally act in certain situations. I realized I couldn't live in the environment I was in and felt my health was inconveniencing our marriage. My oncologist was also concerned that having **chronic stress** could further weaken my immune system which would in turn promote the growth and metastasis of tumors. Four days before starting radiation, I separated from my husband and moved into my own apartment.

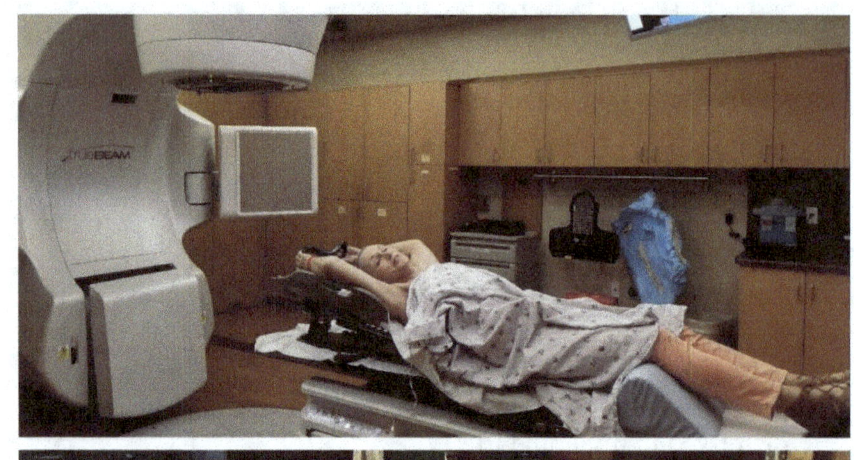

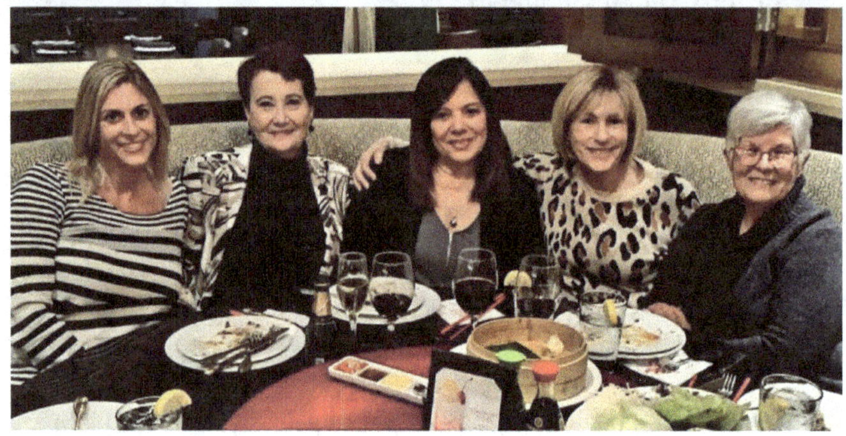

October 30th - Final radiation & celebration!

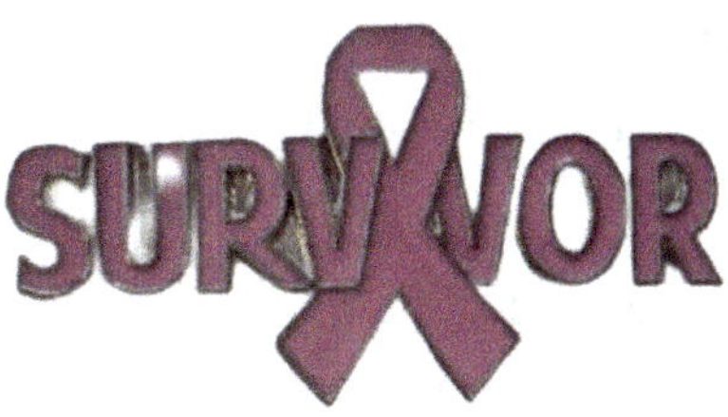

"Difficult roads often lead to beautiful destinations."
Zig Ziglar

The middle of August I had another CAT scan that helped the radiation oncologist locate the treatment area and the surrounding normal tissue. I then had my initial consult at Kaiser Rancho Cordova where my radiologist, Dr. Mahesh Chandra Pant, explained the necessity for these treatments, mainly because of the ratio of positive lymph nodes found. He also mentioned that I would be put on a medicine for the next five to ten years to keep the cancer at bay. It was during this meeting I was reminded of the severity of being a Stage 3A - patient and the importance in following all treatment that was prescribed. It had now been over seven months since my initial diagnosis. I didn't dwell on what the future would hold concerning my breast cancer. I assumed that once I went through all stages of treatment, my life would resume as before.

I think we surprise ourselves in what we can accomplish when we feel our well-being is at stake. In my mind it was a matter of life and death if I stayed in my home as I was feeling extreme stress. Also my marriage wouldn't have a chance in surviving. I mentioned earlier that we were only married three years before the diagnosis and this was unchartered territory for the both of us. Until faced with this situation it is hard to predict how one would act. I think our intentions were to make

71

it through this crisis with our relationship intact - life had another road for me to take.

I still don't know how I coordinated my move. My faith has always carried me through many trials and this one was no exception. I didn't want to involve my family and friends in packing and moving me out. September 21st, I left the property taking just the bare necessities in the hopes that this was only going to be temporary. I knew of a lady who had a pickup and called on her services to help. She and her brother loaded up the truck and moved me to my new apartment. Even now I don't know where I found the strength to accomplish this feat. I settled in, and almost immediately began my daily radiation routine – 3:00 p.m. Monday through Friday for five weeks.

I could finally see the finish line; five weeks to go. By this time I was no longer bald, as my hair had begun growing during my last month of chemotherapy. There were tufts of gray hair coming through on my scalp and some of my eyebrows started to form.

Several friends accompanied me to the first session, September 25th, as they were interested in my procedure and to be of support. I underwent External Beam Radiation Therapy (EBRT) a machine that directs radiation directly to the cancer areas. It is a local treatment that precisely targeted my breast and under my right arm where the lymph nodes were removed. The whole procedure took about 15 minutes with minimal side effects. There was no pain involved, just the discomfort of lying still and hearing the whirr of the machine. It was an odd sensation thinking my body would be radioactive, which it definitely was not. My chest did become very red and itchy but the application of two types of cream; Aquaphor and Medihoney helped in soothing my skin and minimizing any discoloration I had. My treatment would leave me tired but not sickly and I was able to drive myself to all subsequent appointments.

As at my previous treatments, the personnel were so friendly and I felt the assurance of being well taken care of. I also met some of the same patients that were undergoing their own procedure. The protocol was consistent: go into a changing room similar to that of a gym, put on a dressing gown, and nervously wait. I then was escorted through the control room which had television screens to monitor me and the switch that turns on the machine that delivers the radiation. I felt at ease because everything was explained to me. I was then helped onto the table and positioned correctly for the procedure.

 Once I became accustomed to the radiation, my energy level did increase. I spent most of my time reading, walking sometimes up to two miles daily, and resting after treatment. I even tried my hand at learning the ukulele. Mainly I was just looking forward to the end of treatment. Finally, Wednesday, October 30th, arrived. The personnel at Kaiser Radiology congratulated me and wished me all the best. I told them I hoped never to see them again in this environment. I had crossed the finish line…I made it; it was time to really live again!

My daughter, had asked if she could take me out for a celebratory dinner at my favorite restaurant, Fats. I had fully regained my appetite and was ready to party. This would become an annual event as her husband Jeff insisted every October 30th we celebrate with a wonderful meal of my choosing. Unbeknownst, to me she had invited two of my sisters-in-law and a best friend for the occasion. What a festive night it was: great food, plenty of laughter, and surrounded by such wonderful people!

A month later I had another CAT scan and bone density test. I also met with Dr. Balazs Imre (Ernie) Bodai who was head of the Cancer Survivorship Institute. This department offers great support for ongoing recovery. He went over my charts and advised me what I could expect in the near future. He also recommended a healthy eating plan and vitamins that I should take; Calcium and Vitamin D supplements that would help when I started my Zometa infusions. Zometa (Zoledronic acid) is used to prevent problems with the bones and lower the chance of breast cancer returning. I underwent infusions every six months for two years with little to no side effects. My oncologist had also prescribed Letrozole (Femara) which is a type of hormone therapy drug that lowers the levels of the female sex hormone Oestrogen in the body which is known to stimulate some breast cancers to grow. I was told that I would be taking this drug for five to ten years.

I began the first of the Zometa infusions in January 2020; it had been one year since my cancer diagnosis. I had reconciled with my husband and moved back to the property and to be with my beloved Dani. It is difficult to put into words what I was feeling at the time. I know without a doubt that my recovery was made easier because of the many people I have in my life that showered me with such love and care, saying "I am here for you".

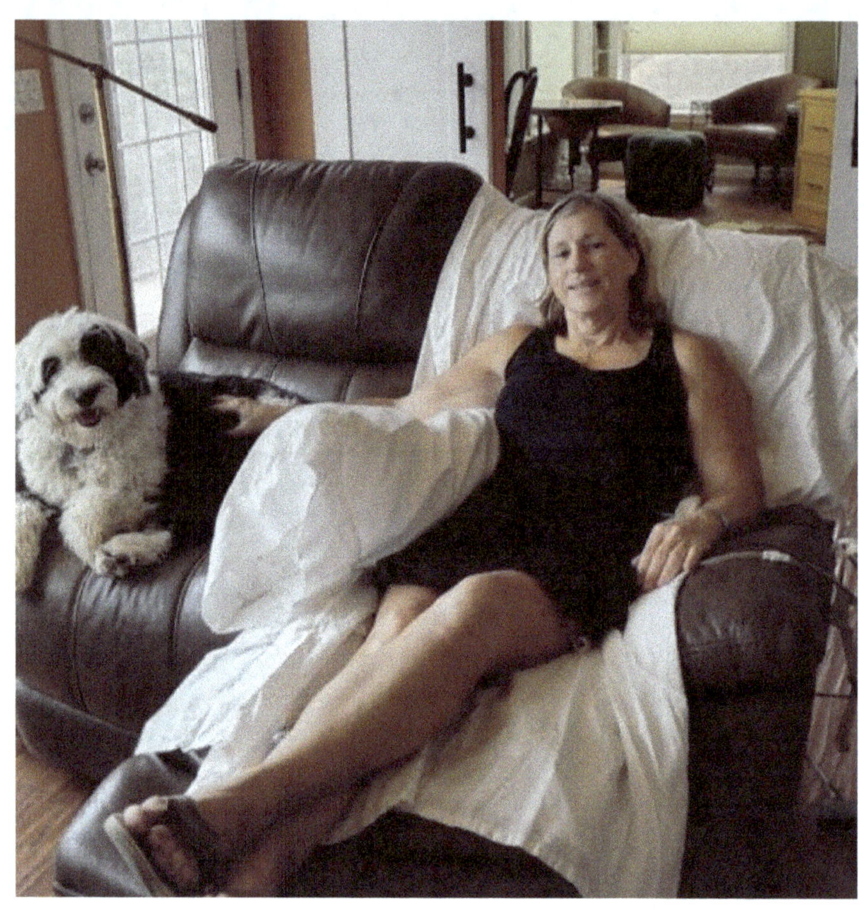

August 2021 – Recovering from reconstruction

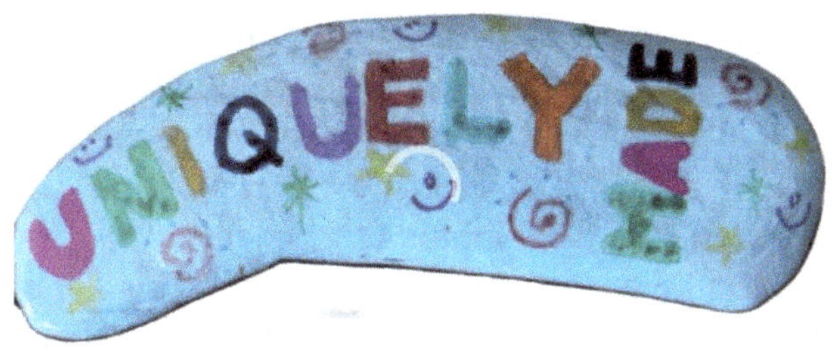

"My breast is all mine; I took it from my stomach."
Stephanie Wolfe Zimmer

I had assumed that I would live the rest of my life without a right breast. The bras and prosthesis that I wore were very comfortable and with clothes on there was no indication that I had only one breast. At my age, (68), I believed I was too old to have reconstruction and had not pursued it. I was busy playing tennis and working part time and never gave it a second thought. One day as I was putting on my bra, one of the hooks broke, which wasn't the first time. It was then that I thought maybe I should look into reconstruction. Sometimes it is the simplest or oddest situation that prompts one to act.

It was March 2021, when I was directed to the Plastic Surgery department at the Kaiser Hospital Morse. It was only a few days before I had a zoom appointment with Dr. Jesus Adrian Garcia. He had familiarized himself with my chart and looked at my bare chest via zoom. In his opinion he didn't think I was a good candidate for expanders with silicon or saline fillers implanted. Due to the intense radiation I underwent, my skin was more translucent and could be in danger of hurting myself with that type of restoration. He did suggest having a Diep (Deep Inferior Epigastric Perforator) flap surgery. This technique was first developed in the 1990's and has become more common in the 2000's.

Within the week, I had an office appointment with Dr. Minh-Bao Mundschenk who would be the attending surgeon. She described in detail the two-part procedure which consisted of the removal of skin, fat tissue and connected blood vessels from my lower abdomen and then transplanting the skin and fat to the chest. She would finish with connecting the blood vessels (arteries and veins) to the chest wall vessels beneath the ribs. Connecting these blood vessels are necessary to keep the tissue healthy. This type of surgery involves the use of special surgical tools and microscopes to tie the blood vessels together. A major benefit to this procedure (unlike other flap surgeries) is that no abdominal muscles are removed. Generally, the surgery is around 4 – 6 hours (for one breast) with a 3-day stay in the ICU unit. Every hour a nurse would then check the breast to see that no fat necrosis has developed due to poor blood supply which would then entail another surgery to remove the fat. At that point the reconstruction would be nulled and if, by chance I were to develop cancer in my left breast, I could not have the same type of Diep flap surgery. There are other flap breast reconstruction options such as removing fat from the back, buttocks, or thighs that then could be considered.

With a Diep flap surgery the reconstructed breast(s) will appear more like a natural breast and is permanent. It also will grow and change when your body does. Unlike breast implant surgery where the breast stays the same even if there is a shift in overall body weight, which could lead to asymmetry in the future. Also implants of silicone or saline last around 10 – 15 years before being replaced. Of course, with the Diep flap surgery there is scarring on the abdomen from the hip-to-hip incision and around the newly formed breast. There is very little scarring with implants and it generally fades in time.

Dr. Mundschenk spent over an hour describing in detail the procedure. She assured me that I was a good candidate as I was active and my body had the right amount of fat that would create a desirable breast. I thought there are some positives to not being "skinny". She told me if I was underweight and had too low of body fat I would have to actually gain some. Also, if there is too much, that could also cause problems. I had so much support from my girlfriends that they unselfishly offered to sacrifice their own body fat to me. Unfortunately only identical twin sisters can be fat donors. Darn!!

I was also told that months after the original surgery I could undergo fat grafting. This procedure is considered a "touch up" to the breast to fix any shape abnormalities and to make alterations that would look more like my other breast. Fat is removed by liposuction without skin, muscle or other tissue and injected into the newly formed breast. At the same time, fat can also be inserted into the other breast if needed for appearance sake. I could also have a nipple created where the surgeon would make a small incision while forming the surrounding tissue into the shape of a nipple. Later the areola can be created by tattooing. With all the information given, I opted for the more invasive surgery with the excitement that my breast cancer journey would soon be complete.

From my initial consultation in March until my surgery, August 16th, 2021, I underwent another CAT scan, extensive blood work, and several pre-op appointments to discuss what I may expect. My operation was shorter than expected - five hours. I was then transported to the recovery room. Because there was a high amount of Covid patients, I never did make it to the ICU. Upon awakening, I was in great spirits. I actually felt like I could get up and start walking. Of course, the first night I wasn't allowed to. I was monitored hourly to check for necrosis. My procedure had been so successful; I was discharged after only a two-night stay.

When I was released from the hospital, I came home with tubes in my chest and abdomen and was fitted with a post-surgery garment. I spent several nights on the recliner as that was more comfortable and I had minimal pain. Dani was by my side the whole time, with Nick as my primary caregiver. After one week I could finally wash my hair.

By the middle of September I was back to walking and playing a little tennis. In the beginning of January 2021 I had signed up for the California International Marathon (CIM) that was held in December. I had participated in the event when I was 39, 49, 59 and I was to turn 69 in November. Unfortunately, I could not get a refund so I thought why not just try to do the 26.2 mile course. My training consisted of playing more tennis in October and November. I had my 3 ½ month checkup December 3rd, and Dr. Mundschenk said I could resume all of my prior activities. I did not tell her that I was planning on doing the marathon two days later.

The morning of the 5th I anxiously awaited the start of the race. It was apparent after a quarter of a mile of jogging that my breast and abdomen would not withstand the jarring. I told myself that I could just walk the rest of the way. After all it was only 26.2 miles. Around the ten-mile mark I came across two ladies who were participating in their first marathon. We actually encouraged each other and crossed the finish line under seven hours (which was their goal), and beat out the remaining four runners. I truly felt that was my best marathon ever. I fulfilled my goal; I had completed the course.

It was April 15th 2022, and I was to undergo my fat grafting procedure. This was done at a Kaiser Outpatient center with Dr. Mundschenk. The surgery went well and I was able to go home the same day. Liposuction was done on my inner thighs and the fat inserted into my right reconstructed breast and a little into the left one. Dr. Mundschenk also created a nipple on my right breast with surrounding excessive skin. Unfortunately, overtime the nipple did recede. I also had my port removed as my Zometa infusions had been completed and there was no need to keep it since I was cancer free. I was put on a waiting list to have a tattoo placed on my reconstructed breast.

Fast forward to March 2024, when to my surprise I received a call from the Kaiser Plastic Surgery department informing me I could finally get my tattoo. I had actually forgot about it and almost declined the appointment. I thought what the heck, this would be an additional picture for my book. On May 7th, 2024, at the Kaiser Plastic Surgery department, my journey ended. I was overwhelmed with the fantastic job that Ashley Flowers, RN did in enhancing my nipple and tattooing the surrounding area to create the areola. Afterwards, looking at my chest, it was almost like I never had cancer. Except for the slight scarring over my right breast, I appear whole.

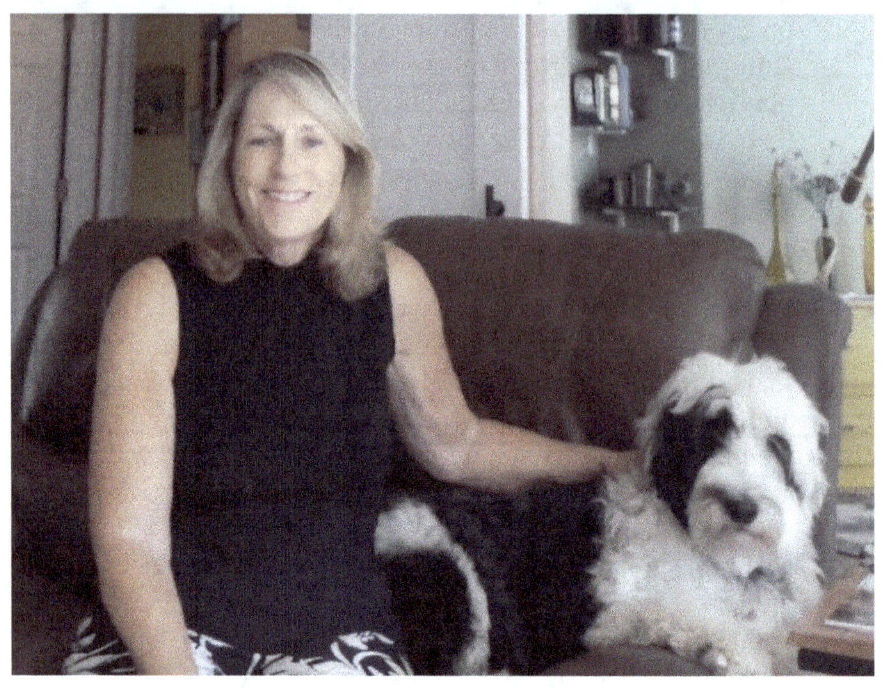

Thank you Dani for accompaning me on this journey!

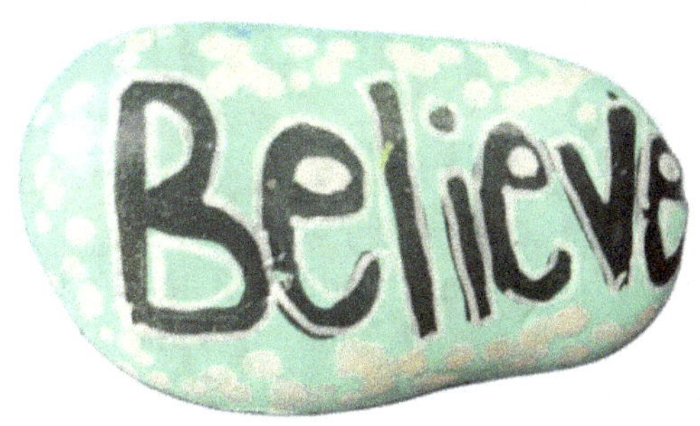

"What lies behind you and what lies in front of you pales in comparison to what lies inside of you."
Ralph Waldo Emerson

From January 10th, 2019, to May 7th, 2024, my medical journey began and ended. As of this writing, I am cancer free and praise the Lord for carrying me through the past, present, and whatever is in my future. This is my story, nothing special, but it has allowed me to process my feelings. Having cancer has changed me in a several ways; I have more empathy towards others going through their health battles. I also realize the importance of being surrounded by the people who love, value, and believe in me. I want to encourage others facing this dreaded disease – don't focus on statistics. Your journey is unique and only God knows your outcome.

I have been fortunate with new treatments and medication not to have suffered like many in the past. When I was first diagnosed, I wanted to hear stories from other breast cancer patients and to see pictures of the different stages they went through. I wrote *Dare to Dream - Again* in the style that I could relate to. I have been given the opportunity to continue

to dream again; maybe hike the Camino Frances in northern
Spain?

It has been said by a former cancer survivor, "You have to
figure out your own way to deal with this diagnosis. You learn
about yourself, what you are made of. This can be
extraordinary and you want to share this and help others who
go through the same thing." [29]

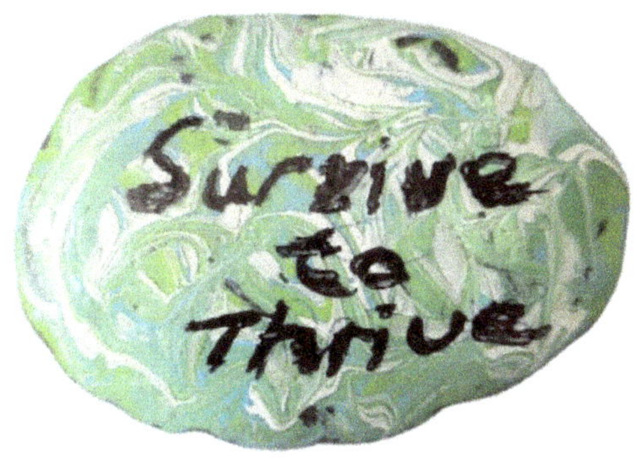

"Every picture tells a story."
Author - Unknown

I am very fortunate to have a loving family and an incredible network of friends. I wanted to be able to look back and remember those who were there to support me. There were many more family members and friends that aren't pictured, but are no less important.

I remember looking in the mirror and saying out loud "That is not me"! It wasn't so much about losing all my hair; that was predictable. I couldn't believe how my hair was growing back. I had to remember, I am a survivor so any hair style is a blessing. Also, shaving my legs now is easier, as not all of that hair came back. It is tricky though, to shave under my right arm as it is numb from the lymph nodes being removed.

After my mastectomy I was curious how my reaction would be when I looked at my chest. My immediate thought was, at least the cancer is cut out and I have a chance for survival. After radiation treatment I was fine to live the rest of my life with a prosthesis for a breast. When I made the decision for reconstruction I never imagined my chest could look normal.

Having Dani join our family truly was a blessing. Raising a puppy with all of its challenges, took some of the focus off of me. I am so fortunate to have had her by my side and the incredible love that only a pet can give.

"Try to be a rainbow in someone's cloud."
Maya Angelo

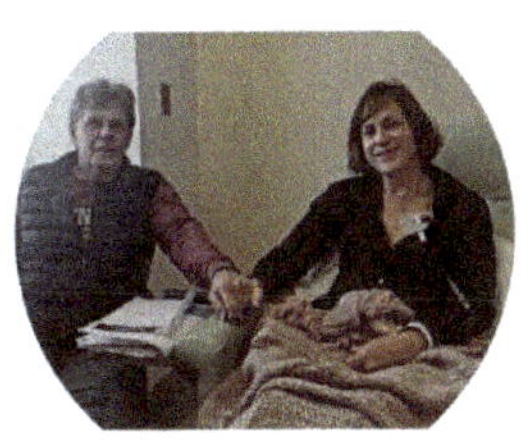

Nick 1st chemo

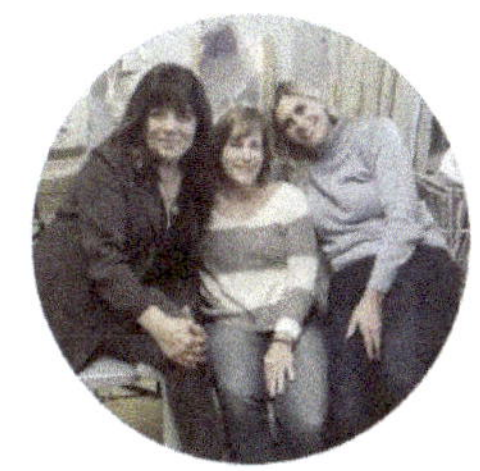

Grace & Shannon

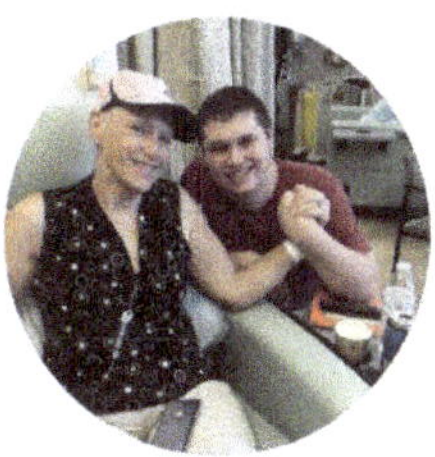

Grandson Tyler

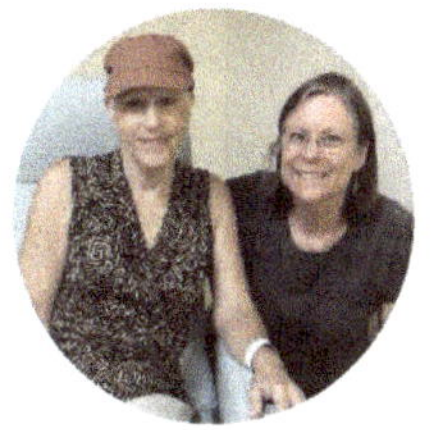

Robin

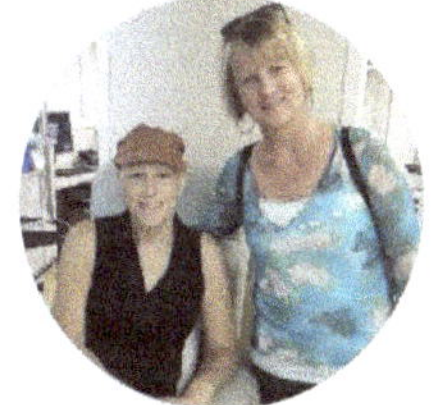

Cindy

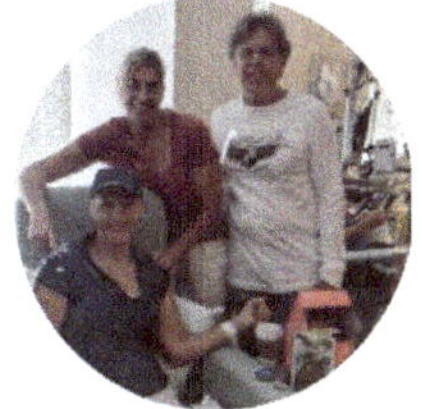

Final chemo

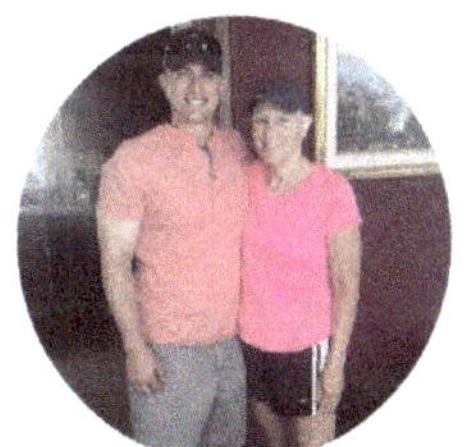

Jason

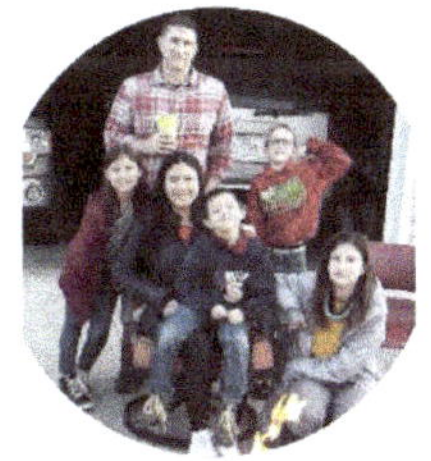

Jason, Emy
Savannah, Jayme
Roy & Jason Jr.

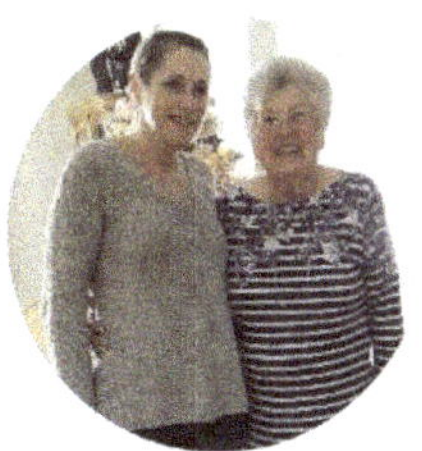

Aunt Maxine

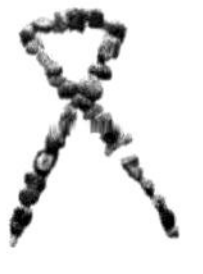

Women's Hair Loss Project

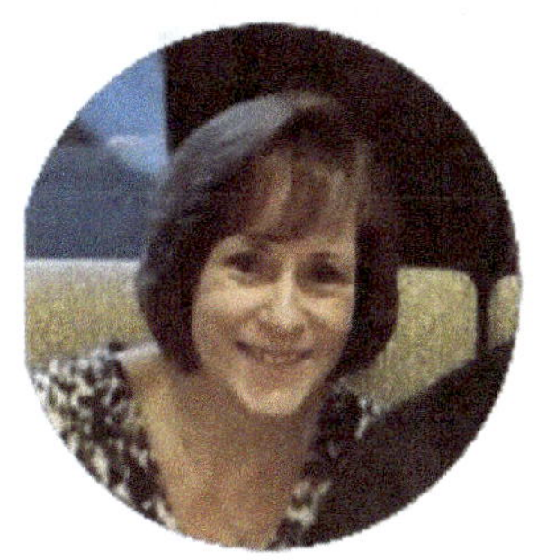

January before lumpectomy

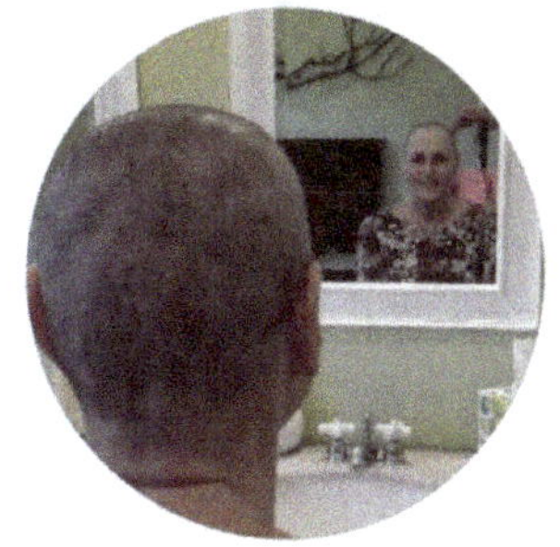

April buzz cut

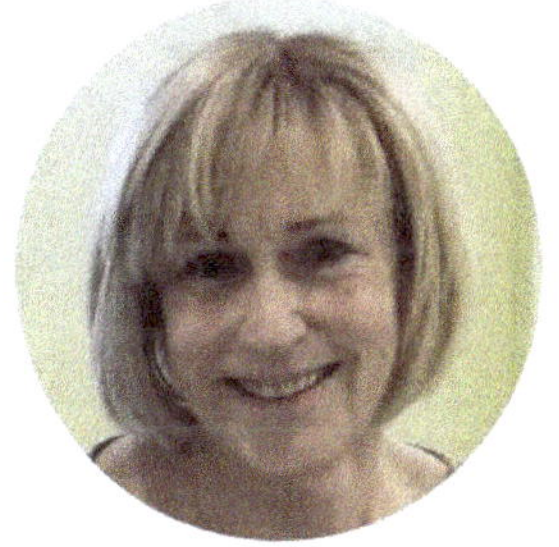

Cindy's wig

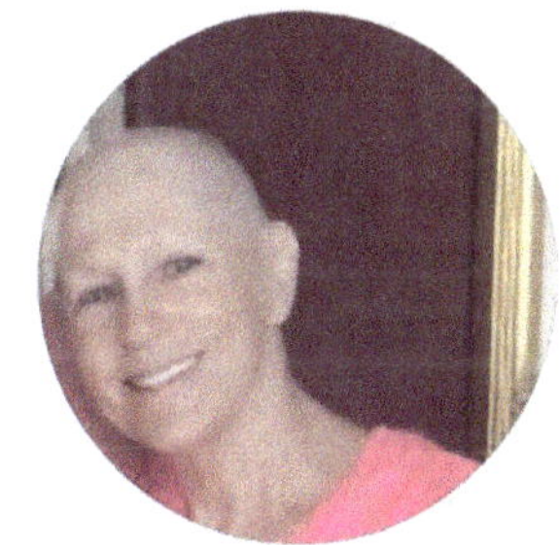

July more chemo

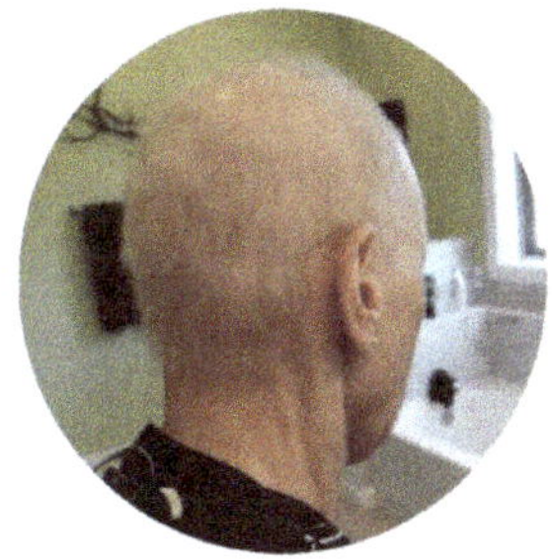

Early September

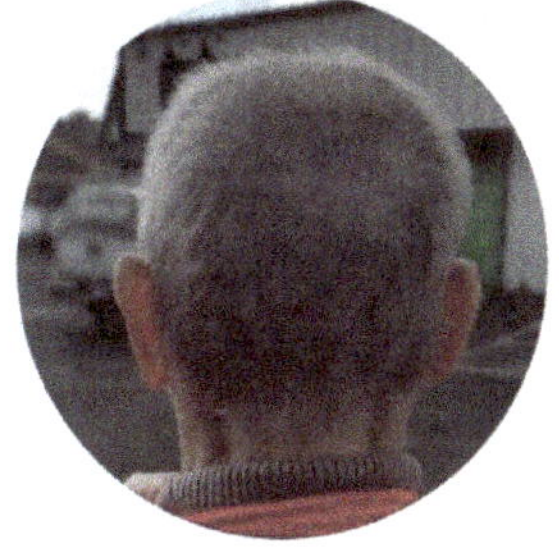

Early October

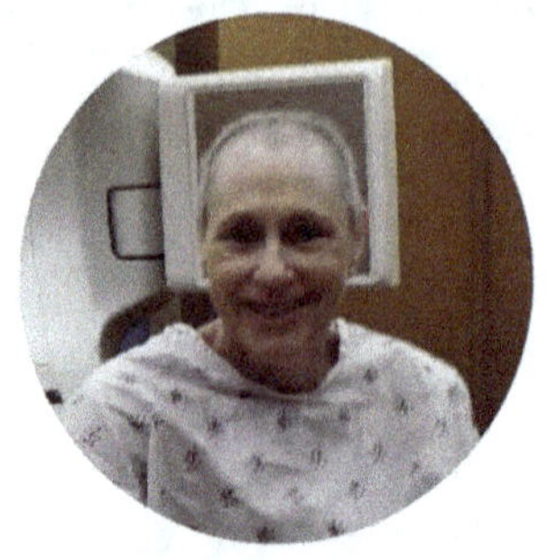

October 30th last radiation

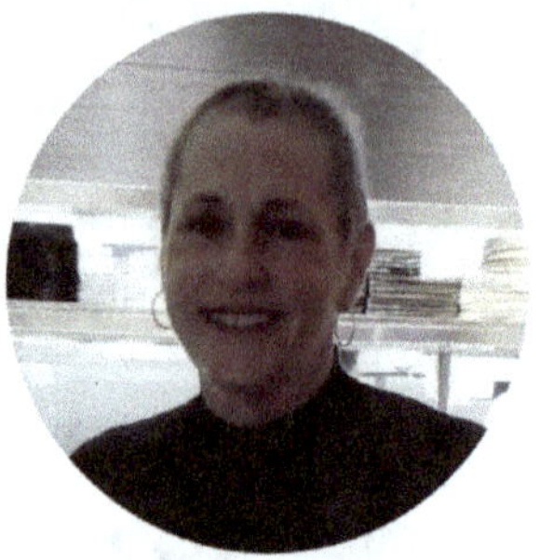

November birthday

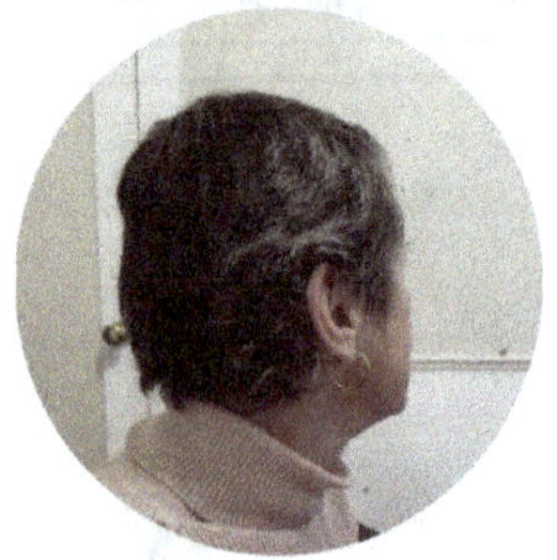

2020 last of January

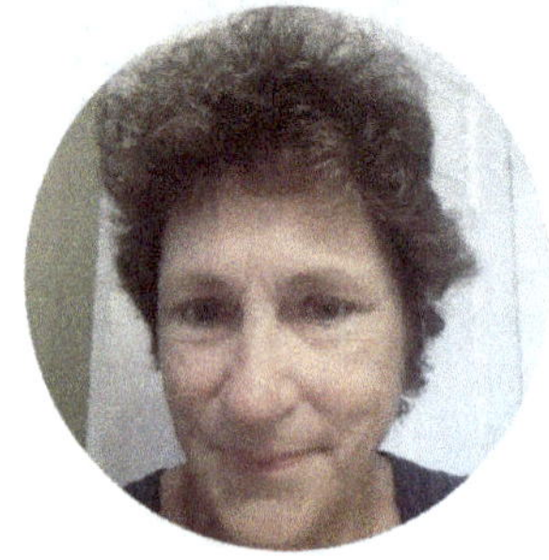

April so fuzzy

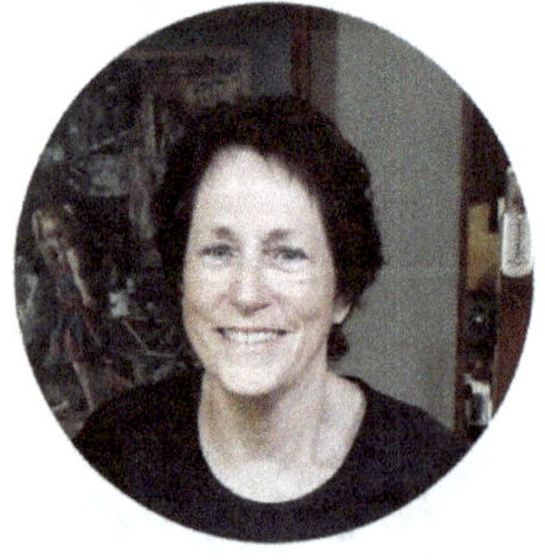

May erased the gray

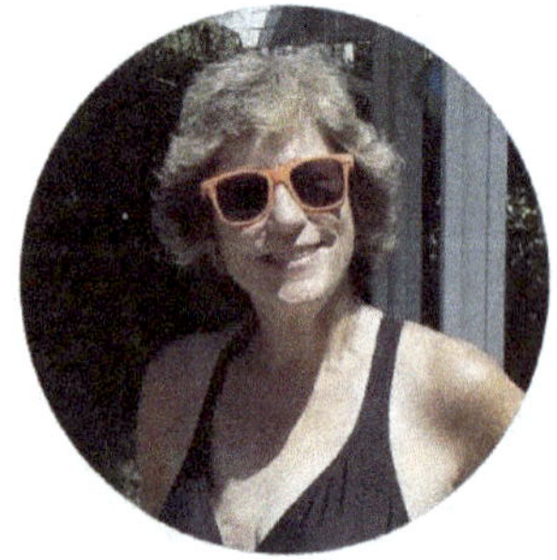

August sunbleached

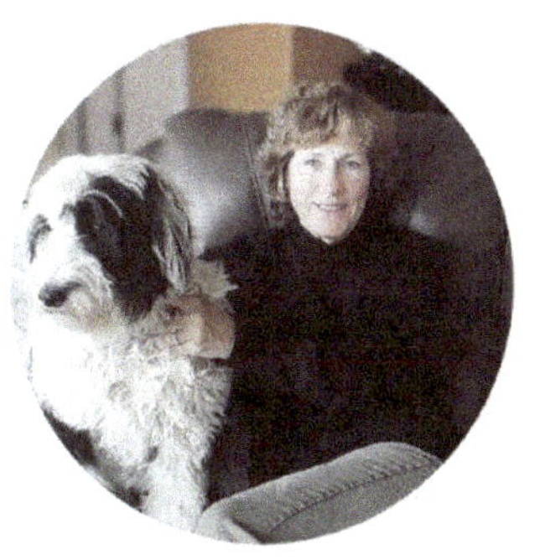

September still wavy

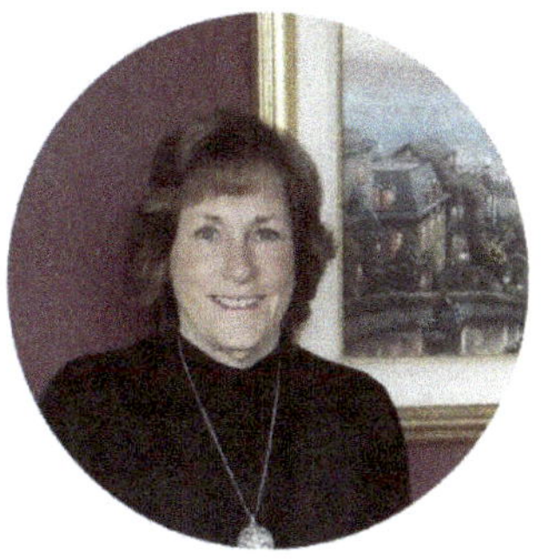

October 2020 one year later

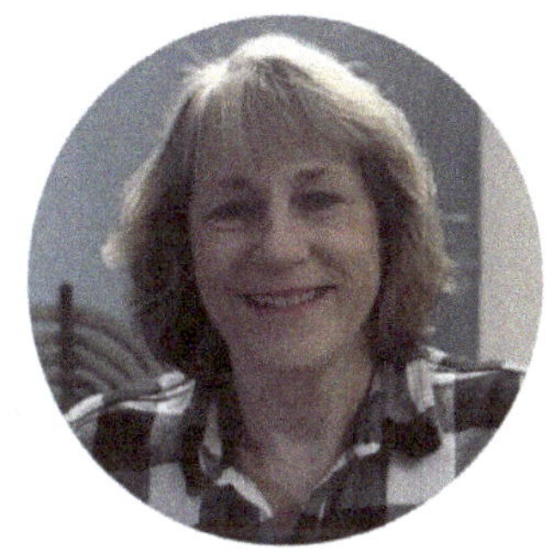

October 2022 back to normal

"My relationship with my body has changed. I used to consider it as a servant who should obey, function, give pleasure. In sickness, you realise that you are not the boss. It is the other way around."

Federico Fellini

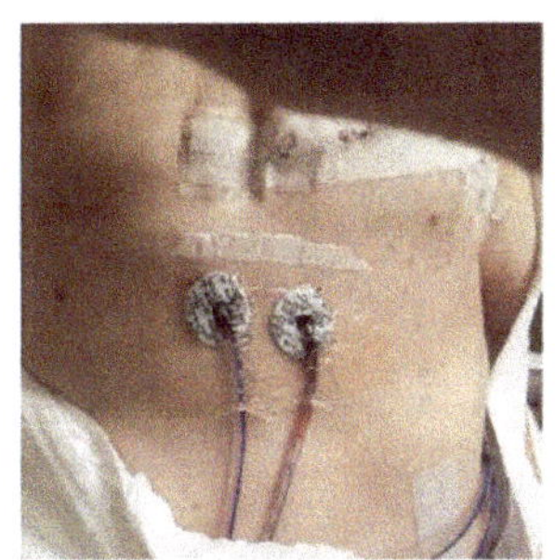

2019 Mastectomy

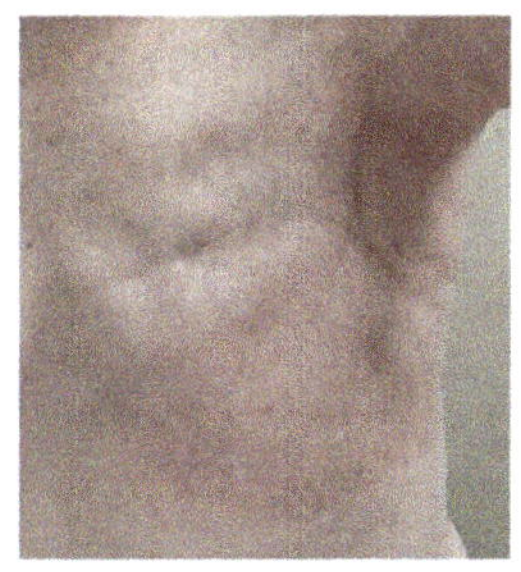

Final radiation

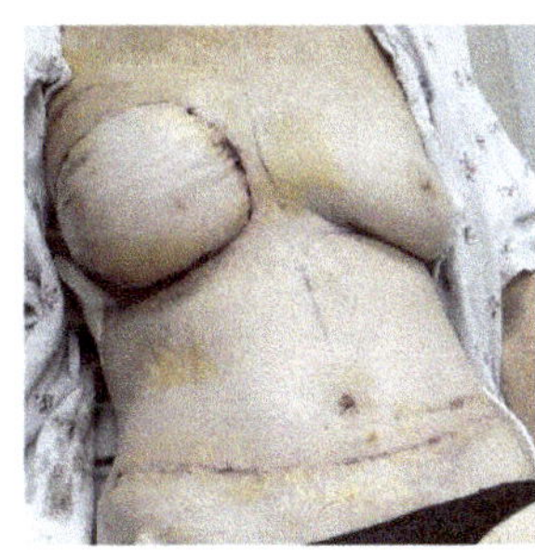

2021 Reconstruction

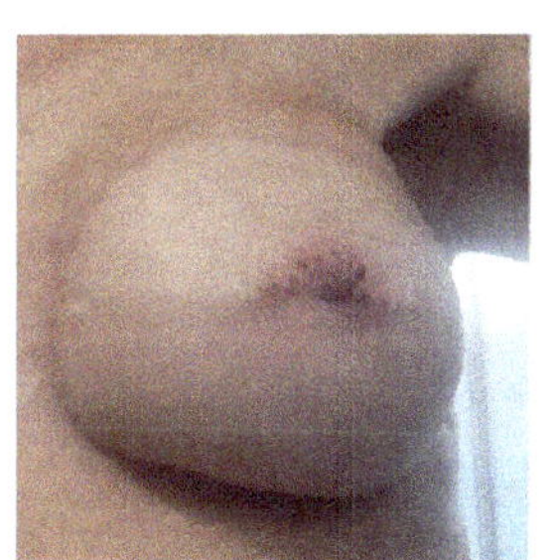

2022 nipple created

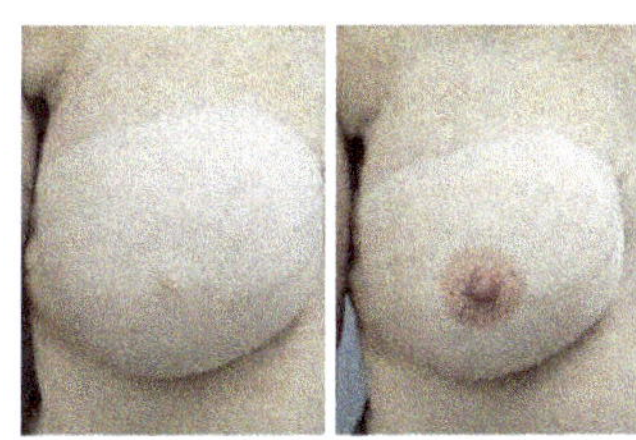

May 2024 before & after tattoo

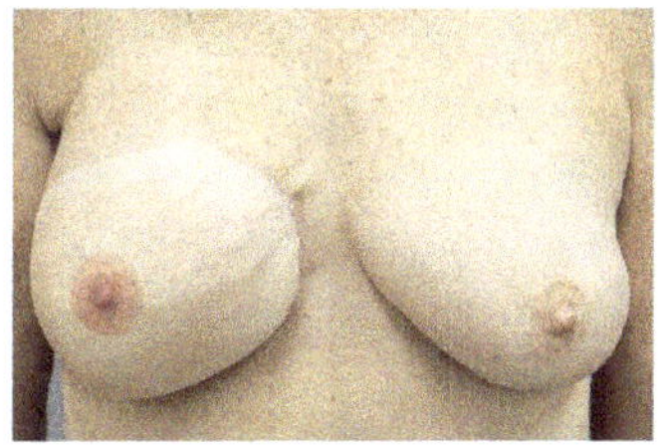

May 7th made whole

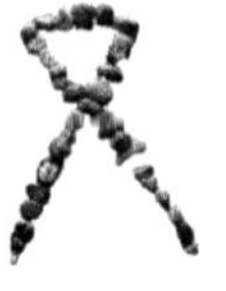

94

"No one loves you as unconditionally as your beloved pet."
Cynthia Dobesh

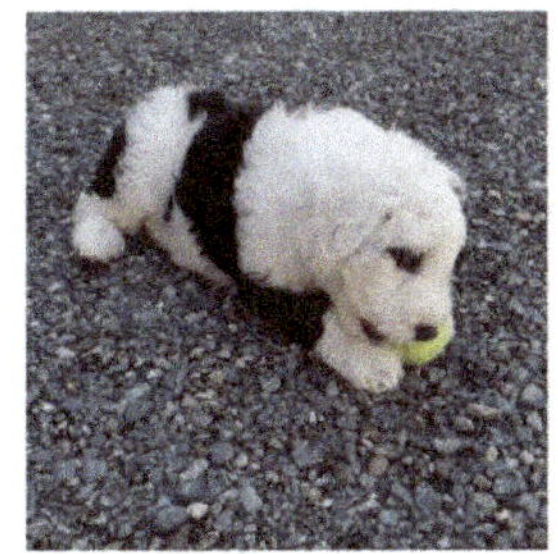

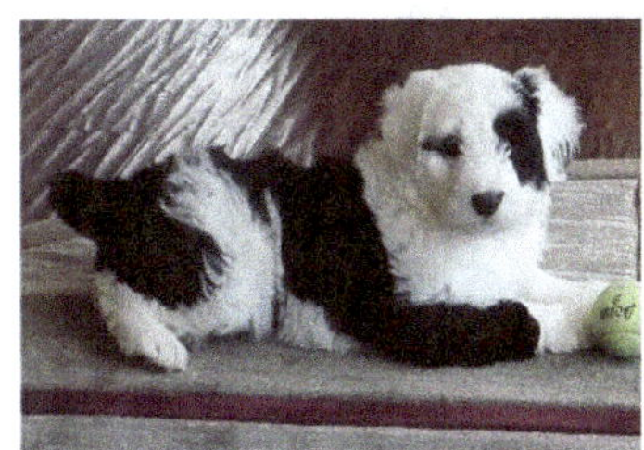

Dani born November 8th 2018

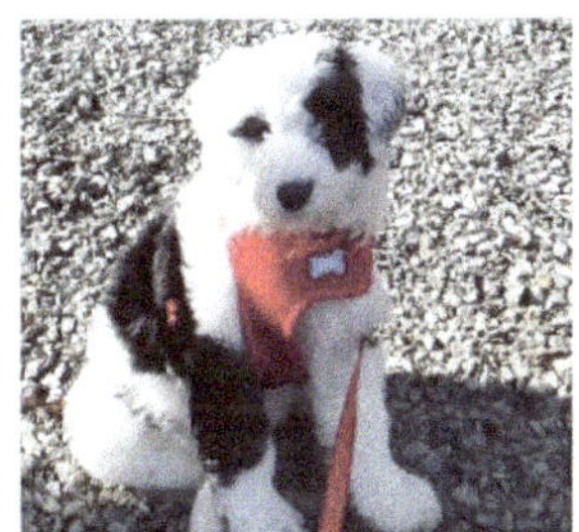

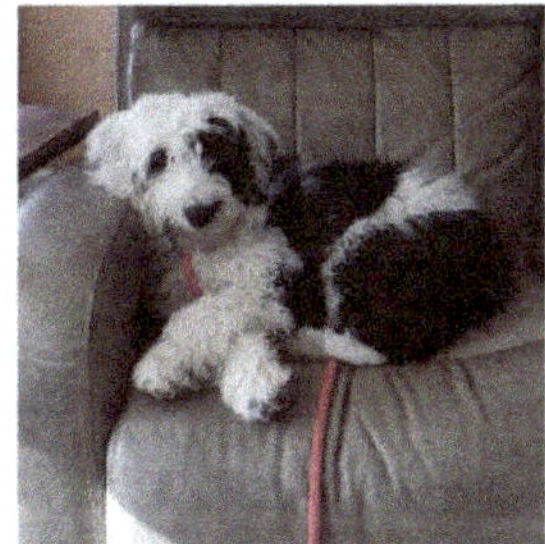

Growing cuter and spoiled

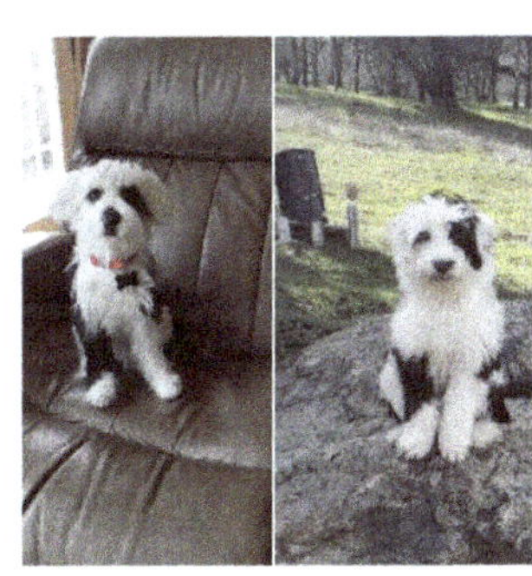

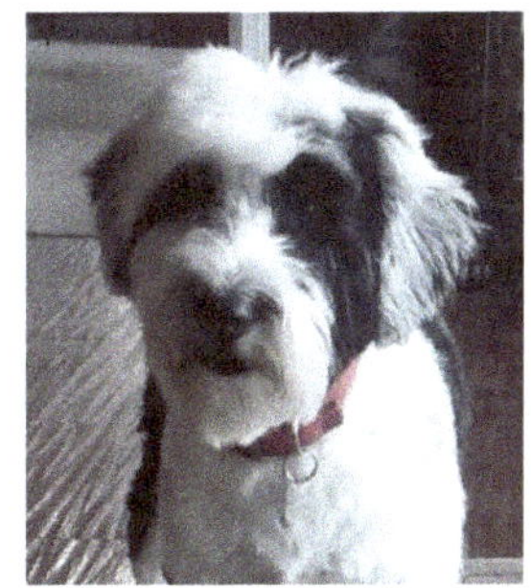

Duplicate Dani - shaved for summer

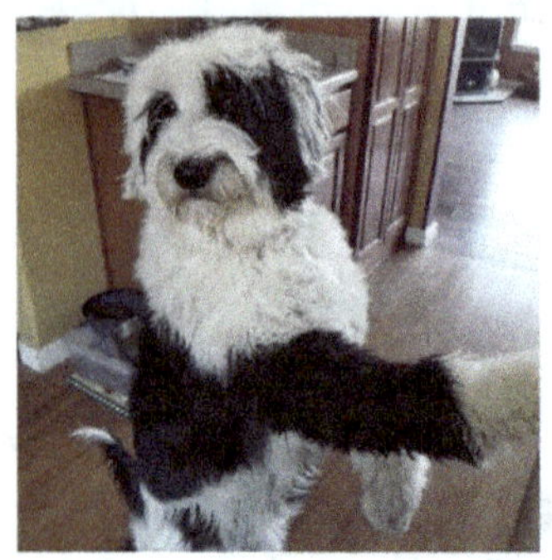 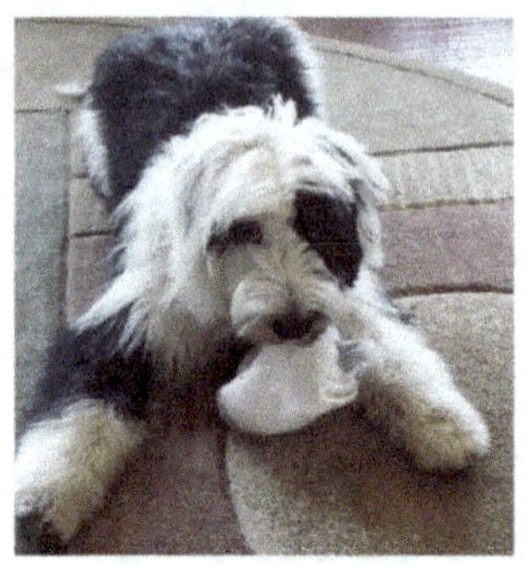

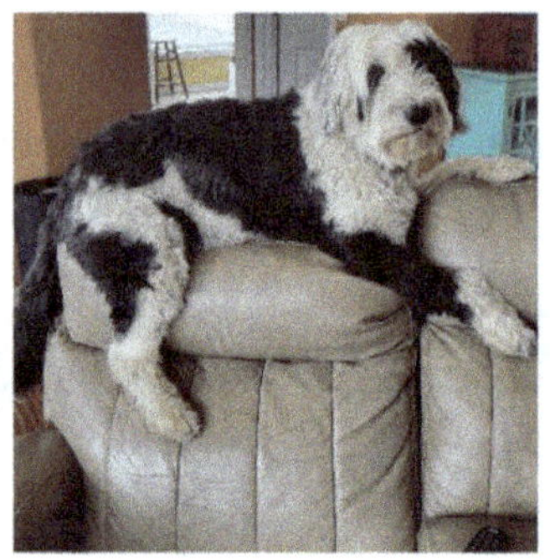

Dani all grown up

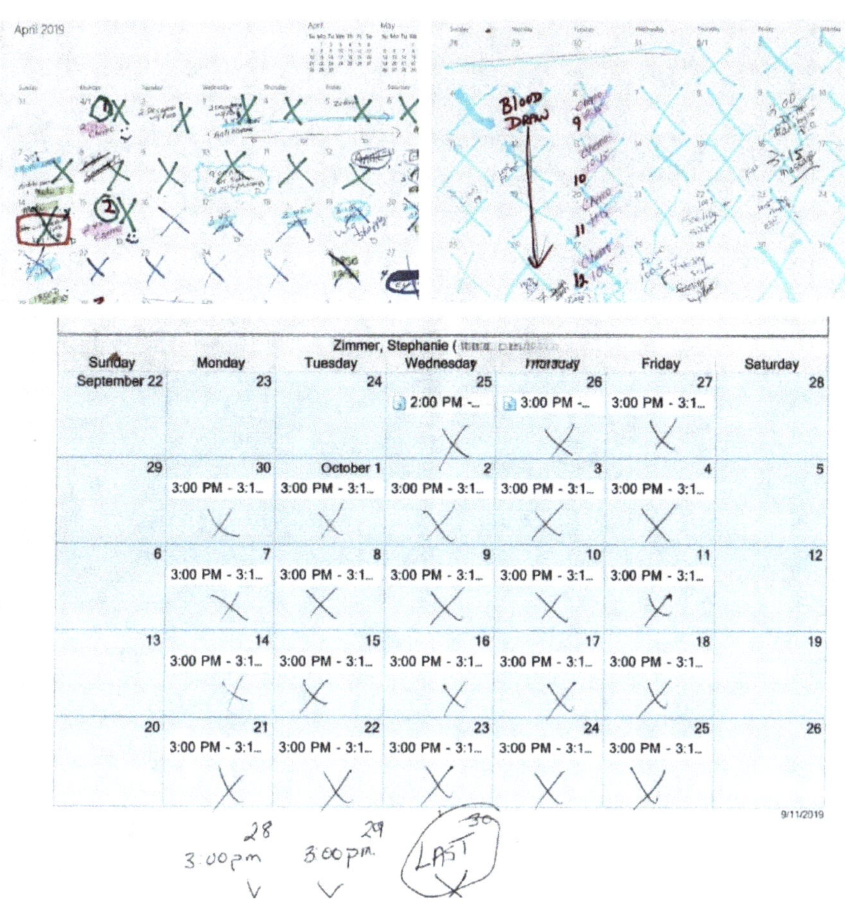

I lived for my X's; finally finished!

Citations

I wrote *Dare to Dream – Again,* over a two-year period. I read quite a bit of information on the history of breast cancer and the accounts of women who battled their disease. I relied on the internet to get most of my data. While taking notes, I did not always record where I acquired my facts; one site would inevitably lead me to another source. I am confident that my citations are reliable and there is no intent on my part to mislead the reader. Any medical terms described in my treatment came from my doctors, their notes, and hospital information packets.

---

[1] From Benjamin Rush to John Adams, 20 September 1811. *Founders Online* National Archives, https://founders.archives.gov/documents/Adams/99-02-02-5687

[2] Olson, JS. *Bathsheba's Breast: Women, Cancer & History:* Essay on Abigail Adams. Baltimore, MD: The Johns Hopkins University Press; 2002, pg. 39.

[3] Jimenez, RE. *"A Monument to suffering and to patience": The harrowing journey of Nabby Adams through Breast Cancer.* 2023, *Journal of Medical Biography*; Vol. 31(2): 133-142.

[4] Olson, JS. *Bathsheba's Breast:* 2002, pg.40.

[5] John Collins Warren, https://g.co/kgs/XdBAvnS

[6] Olson, JS. *Bathsheba's Breast*: 2002, pg.41.

[7] Jimenez, RE. *"A Monument to suffering and to patience"*: 2023, pg. 141.

[8] Letters of Note, https://www.lettersofnote.com/2012/02/deep-sickness-seized-me.html

[9] Life, Death and Surgery through a lens,
https://www.sterileeye.com/2012/02/29/a-mastectomy-in-1855

[10] Letters of Note, 2012.

[11] From Herodotus (485 – 430 BC). Yan SH. *An early history of human breast cancer: West meets East* .Chin J Cancer. 2013 Sep; v32(9). National Library of Medicine.

[12] Yan SH. *An early history of human breast cancer: West meets East.* Chin J Cancer. 2013; v32(9). National Library of Medicine.

[13] Mahmoud A. *Historic, Present, and Future Perspectives on Breast Cancer in Egypt.* August 25, 2021. The ASCO Post.

[14] Freeman MD, Gopman JM, Salzberg CA. *The evolution of mastectomy surgical technique: from mutilation to medicine.* Gland Surg 2018;7(3):308-315. doi:10.21037/gs.2017.09.07.

[15] *Understanding What Cancer is: Ancient Times to Present.* American Cancer Society
https://www.cancer.org/cancer/understanding-cancer/history-of-cancer/what-is-cancer.html

[16] Freeman MD, Gopman JM, Salzberg CA. *The evolution of mastectomy surgical technique.* 2018.

[17] Mandal, Ananya. (2019, February 26). *History of Breast Cancer.* News-Medical. Retrieved on September 05, 2024 from
https://www-medical.net/health/History-of-Breast-Cancer.aspx

[18] Mandal, Ananya. (2019, February 26). *History of Breast Cancer.*

[19] Freeman MD, Gopman JM, Salzberg CA. *The evolution of mastectomy surgical technique.* 2018.

[20] Breast cancer research, dies at 101 – University of Pittsburgh
https://www.pitt.edu/pittwire/features-articles/bernard-fisher-md-pioneer-breast-cancer-research-dies-101

[21] *History of Cancer Treatments: Chemotherapy.* American Cancer Society https://www.cancer.org/cancer/understanding-cancer/history-of-cancer/cancer-treatment-chemo.html

[22] Mandal, Ananya. (2019, February 26). *History of Breast Cancer.*

[23] Brevard Health Alliance (2019, October 17). *A Brief History of Breast Cancer Awareness Month* https://www.brevardhealth.org/blog/a-brief-history-of-breast-cancer-awareness-month/

[24] Breast Cancer Action. In Memoriam: *Charlotte Haley, Creator of the First (Peach) Breast Cancer Ribbon* https://www.bcaction.org/in-memoriam-charlotte-haley-creator-of-the-first-peach-breast-cancer-ribbon/

[25] Fernandez, SM. (reprinted from MAMM, June/July 1998) Breast Cancer Action. *History of the Pink Ribbon; Pretty in Pink* https://www.bcaction.org/about-think-before-you-pink/resources/history-of-the-pink-ribbon/

[26] Breast Cancer Foundation - Susan G. Komen https://www.komen.org/milestones.pdf

[27] Breast Cancer Foundation - Susan G. Komen https://www/komen.org/uploadedfiles/content_binaries/the_pink-ribbon_ story.pdf

[28] Breast Cancer Statistics | *How Common is Breast Cancer?* | American Cancer Society https://www.cancer.org/cancer/types/breast-cancer/about/how-common-is-breast-cancer.html

[29] Cancer survivors day attendee (2012) Hopeful Quotes|Sharing Hope|University of Michigan Rogel Cancer Center https://www.rogelcancercenter.org/living-with-cancer/sharing-hope/hopeful-quotes#

9798339780038